SISTERS

CRITICAL ACCLAIM FOR "SISTERS"

"A tender and witty book"   — Mary Kenny, *Irish Press*

"A brave, clear-eyed and perceptive account of one woman's emergence to being truly herself."
                    — Gemma Hussey, *Evening Press*

"An important historic document that should be read and kept by every woman."   — Clare Boylan, *Image*

"Compulsive reading. She is funny, honest, compassionate and uncompromisingly mature."
                    — Kate Cruise O'Brien, *Irish Press*

"A book for women which every man living with an Irish woman should read."
                    — Ronit Lentin, *Sunday Independent*

"Moving, memorable and timely."
                    — Monica Barnes, *National Democrat*

SISTERS

JUNE
LEVINE

**WARD
RIVER
PRESS**

First published 1982 by
Ward River Press Ltd.,
Knocksedan House,
Swords, Co. Dublin, Ireland
Revised and reprinted 1983 and 1985

© June Levine, 1982

ISBN 0 907085 43 1

Cover design by Steven Hope
Typeset by Inset Ltd.,
171 Drimnagh Road, Dublin 12.
Printed by Mount Salus Press Limited,
Tritonville Road, Dublin 4.

For Diane, my daughter, in sisterhood

ACKNOWLEDGEMENTS

I wish to thank, most warmly, those who helped me in the writing of this book, whether with their memories, interviews or encouragement. Thanks to Mary Sheerin for turning on my memory, to Mary Kenny for lending me her scrap book, to Roisin Conroy for letting me plough through the files of Irish Feminist Information, and to Pat Brennan for her article about the Irish Women's Movement in *Magill*. My thanks to Clare Boylan, Máirín Johnston, Margaret Gaj, Nell McCafferty, Nuala Fennell TD, Mary Maher, Rosita Sweetman, Colette O'Neill, Janet Martin, Maura O'Dea, Liz McWeeney, Celine Henry, Bairbre Madden Reddy. Thanks to Andrew Whittaker, Vincent Kenny, Kevin Clear and editor Cormac Ó Cuilleanáin. A special thanks to Ivor Browne and ultimately to my beloved "Babuji". Apologies to those people who should have been mentioned in the text and aren't; some names, however, have been altered or concealed to avoid embarrassment to individuals.

June Levine

CONTENTS

1
SISTER

She's like a sister to me now, that female who was me, exasperating when she edges me aside, and interferes with the way I want to be now, stirring up old habits born of the old rules, tricks to pull me down, leave nothing gained. Still, I understand and accept her; after all, sisterhood is powerful. I'm quite fond of that woman who was me. God, she was hard to live with, hard to know, hard to convince, but she was young, beautiful, vivacious, believing that those assets would fulfil the myth of womanhood prized ...

She wasn't stupid, just naive — courage headed in the direction of hopelessness. She cost me dearly. Together, entangled, we almost destroyed ourselves in hiding from each other. Now we try to keep one another at bay most of the time, getting along OK, and when she creeps up out from under my guard, I slap her down. Her more subtle intrusions bring me out in itchy spots. One such spot on my right cheek, looking pre-menstrual, heralds the fact that she's up to something. My cheek erupts before I realise I'm under attack. "For Christ's sake," I ask her in the mirror, "what are you up to now?" Sometimes it takes weeks for her answer to whisper to the surface, weeks of an angry spot on my face. Between myself and that other one, there will be conflict to the end. I'm aware that sometimes I spite her, not doing what I want to do because I think it's her choice, her whispering. Pathetic, pleasing, winning, smiling, agonised temporarily by the rejection she brings on herself and then smiling again, into the song and dance routine.

Will we always watch each other? I keep a conscious eye on her; her view of me is more sporadic. Shock makes her surface. I'm buttering up some man and she smiles approvingly, making me feel a traitor to myself ... I become cold, distant, impatient to remove myself elsewhere. Or I am striding past a shop window, engrossed in thought, and I feel her shocked by what she sees. There I am, looking just like me, a middle-aged woman, nothing fantasised, comfortable clothes, naked face, shoes for walking. Still, the knowledge that she wouldn't be caught dead like that makes me pull in my stomach. She causes me an uneasy moment, making me remember how we were. One of these days I'll give her something to gasp about. I'll go somewhere formal 'midst pomp and paint and posturing and I'll be *comfortable,* easy clothes, friendly shoes, braless because I will have learned to accept that floppy feeling as part of myself, hair greying, eyes undefined, broken veins and scars and blotches innocent of that tawny beige cream that smoothed my skin the same as butter on bread. And if I laugh or cry there'll be no little black streams down my cheeks.

Tears. I remember the first time I cried woman tears. Was I five years old? It was when I learned my mother had a different name from my father and me and my two brothers. No, I might have been seven. My mother's name was McMahon but she couldn't be called that anymore because she was married. So my mother had to pretend, I thought. Pretend to be like my father. Did mothers have to pretend to be one of the family? Were they not really? Did they just have to take a new name when they came to work in a family and then when all the work was done they'd get to be themselves again? Not have to pretend anymore? When we were all grown up could my mother get her name back again? "No, no," Nanny, my mother's mother, told me, "you have such a notion." Mammy would never be called McMahon again, now she was Muriel Levine. Fathers earn the few shillings, she explained, and

were the boss of the family so everybody was called by the name they had, well, so as not to mix up Willie the postman. So mothers didn't matter? Nanny looked alarmed. I can see her now, pedalling her sewing machine, guiding the blue organza under the needle: of course mothers matter. Mothers were more important than anybody. Fathers too, but you couldn't manage anyway in the world without a mother, now could you?

I felt panic. I'd ask Willie, I told her, if he'd mind if I kept my own name and he could deliver letters to me. Ah no, love, you could only do that if you wanted to be an old maid and sure that wouldn't be likely and who'd want it? Although, said Nanny, sometimes a body would wonder. Poor Katie had her own name, but sure the creature hadn't much else, only us, no man, no chick or child. Poor Auntie Katie had been Engaged, Nan said. He was a lovely fellow and he went off for to be a soldier and wasn't he killed and Katie never overed it. That's why she was so touchy and cried so much. Her name? Katherine Casey. And yours, Nan, what's your *really* name? Christina Casey, but sure that's water under bridges now. I won't get married at all, Nan, never, you won't have to make me a dress with a veil. I'd rather still be me by my name and not disappear. You can make me another pink dress when I get big. Disappear? Child, where did you get that notion? Who's been putting notions in your head? Disappear, my goodness! Sure isn't your mother gone to Clery's, not disappeared, amn't I here not disappeared? I cried then. Nan was pretending she didn't mind being disappeared. No one to save me. I cried and couldn't stop. I was going to disappear or else have my fella killed in the war and be whingy, crinkly and yellow like Auntie Katie. The tears made my throat ache. Was that the beginning of my departure from myself, the split that formed the two of us, trying to live together?

I did, of course, get married, when I was barely nineteen. Not to have married, even so young, would have been, I realise now, like swimming against a rampaging sea. The tide through which my life was washed swept towards

marriage, inevitably, from the cradle. The self I'd grown into was too fragile, ill-formed, lacking in rôle-models, to prevent the trap snapping. Everything else was just pretend, play, distraction, by the way. The core business of my life was Getting Married. She was hell-bent on that in spite of me. Before I was 16 years old I was working as a cub in the reporters' room of the *Irish Times*. I was "promising," and didn't notice anything amiss in those late 'forties when the lad who was taken on with me took off in another direction, with the men. While he made his way through courts, Dáil and general reporting, I learned the "woman's angle", sales of work, social and personal column, fashion writing even then when paper was scarce, then on to Children's Courts, human interest stories. My "flair" was encouraged to add the bit of femininity the paper needed in the days when it was believed women didn't read papers anyway, but opportunity by-passed me in the way of training. In spite of the system and because, I think, I was a pretty sexually precocious youngster, I got all kinds of help from other reporters. I learned more than I could have done in any school. The more they fussed over me, the more man-mad I became, being chased by one of the bosses at one stage, a man many years older than myself, offering me the kind of opportunity that's recognised as "office harassment" by feminists today. Then, his attentions seemed bliss.

There was, of course, a good biological reason for my obsession with men. They were the opposite sex and they liked me. I didn't have a convent background where I might have been told that boys led to danger or sin. My sexual awareness was not doused in guilt and fear. In fact, nobody ever told me anything at all about boys. I picked up my attitude to men as I went along, mainly from experience of their behaviour. My mother was fifteen years old when I was born, my father eighteen. I can still get in touch with the feeling of their sexuality in the atmosphere when I was a child. I remember them, in my early years, behaving towards each other as you'd expect turned-on teen-agers to behave, touching, smooching, whispering.

Their relationship was pretty stormy and sexually vibrant, and was to form threads in the pattern of my own expectations of heterosexual relationships for many a year to come. Sex education is never, ever, absent from family life. It may be negative, it may be covert or sterile, but it is sex education nonetheless. The child absorbs the atmosphere of the parent's sexuality into her unconscious so that it becomes a part of her own sexuality. In this respect, I've always felt that parents can say what they like to children about sex, but it is what they, the parents, are as sexual beings that matters before all. My parents did not start behaving like middle-aged married people until they were well into grandparenthood, which happened when they were aged thirty-six and thirty-eight years respectively.

Besides always feeling sexy, I realised quite early in life that men ran the world outside the home. They had power and money, but apart from that a woman who couldn't earn their approval was pathetic — left-over, dowdy, second-best. They were the way and the salvation when I was a girl. The way to what, the salvation of what, I did not think out too clearly. But men were an answer. In that context I obviously knew at some level that to marry well was a feminine achievement. One married "up", never "down".

And yet I wasn't consciously aware of sifting wheat from chaff. *She* may have been up to that; I was not. Who to marry, after all? I had so much contempt for all of the young men with whom I spent so much time. The night I became engaged to a Canadian Jewish medical student, I knew I had pulled It off. My father, especially, would be well pleased with me, and he was. So were my Jewish grandparents (the others were dead by now), my aunts, uncles, brothers, sisters, perhaps even my mother. To have done something so right, by accident as I thought, was very exciting. It was wonderful to float around in a cloud of tribute for months until the wedding, feeling approval everywhere, the fulfilment of everyone's expectations.

What, I asked my father, would I do about the job I had got myself in Fleet Street? Ah, forget that nonsense, he said, this was worth more. I never asked how he meant that. Did he really see marriage as such an opportunity for a woman, the ideal for his daughter? Years later, when I got divorced, he advised me: "What you should do now is look for a husband ..." To this day, there is still no greater joy a daughter could give my father than to tell him she was getting married, especially to a nice Jewish boy. Other good news would be pregnancy, a husband achieving something, sons doing well, news of somebody else's daughter getting married. The solid achievement of looking so well that you deserved a good husband came high on his list, as in: "She's a beautiful-looking girl, is there no sign of her getting married?"

"Daddy, she's a surgeon ..."

"You'd think that girl would have lots of fellows after her. Maybe she's too particular."

There was every danger that I might have caused ructions in the family by "marrying out". My father had done precisely that, being the son of an immigrant Jew and my mother the daughter of McMahons from Co. Clare. That was different. It couldn't happen again; there was no reason why it should. Weren't we brought up Jewish? The fact that we were brought up Jewish by a mother who came from a convent school made no difference. We would absorb Judaism; Christianity was not really anything to do with us; and even if some, nay many, Jewish families mightn't like their children to marry into ours, weren't his daughters beautiful girls? As for the boys, there was such a shortage of Jewish boys in Dublin that parents would be proud to get a son-in-law named Levine. In those days before group therapy, marriage counselling and letting it all hang out, my father decided for himself that his family were going to marry Jews: not *finished!* "Finished" didn't mean that that was what we would be if we married "out"; "finished" is a Jewish expression which means "that's all", "the matter's settled" or "nothing more to discuss". It's used to simplify a problem, whether family ructions, the arrangements for an affair (a party involving food, not the other kind of affair) or simply what to serve guests:

chopped liver, chicken soup, brisket, lochen cuggel, followed by lemon sherbet. Finished! So what's to fuss?

Except, of course, our family didn't work out like that. Myself and my sister married Jews. My brothers defected. A good sign, you might say, if Freud's theories can be taken seriously, the girls looking for men like their father, the boys in pursuit of their mother. But it was hard on my father's blood pressure each time it happened. All three married Dublin Catholic girls. Les, the artist who lives in New York, was soon divorced from his first choice and went on to marry a Japanese girl and a Hawaiian, his present wife. He's now a Buddhist priest. I have gone past Judaism and Christianity in latter years to an Eastern form of meditation, with a lingering reliance and fondness for the Blessed Virgin handed to me — it seems like a gift now — by my maternal grandmother.

As a child, I often promised myself that one day I would be a Christian. So much of Judaism I loved, and do to this day, but for me as a child the promises of Jesus Christ surpassed the promises of the Old Testament. Being as many as the grains of sand on the beach didn't grab me, being chosen smacked a bit of being the favourite or the pet and I had reason to know there was a sting in that for someone, the Promised Land seemed far off and I wanted to stay in Ireland anyway, but Jesus, Christmas, Easter and Mary were given to me as forbidden fruit and for years I felt myself to be part of a wonderful secret fairy story.

I hadn't met a Christian boy I wanted to marry by the time I was nineteen, and, although I still loved the Passover and said the Hail Mary, I hadn't made a religious choice. Falling in love with a Jew, a pure-bred, second-generation Russian Jew who had spoken only Yiddish until he went to school, clinched things for me. Hadn't Ruth said: "Whither thou goest ..."? All solved. I needn't make a public declaration of allegiance to Christ and his holy Mother, I needn't hurt my beloved grandfather Nathan or incur the rage of my father. The one time I brought up the subject of religion with my husband he said: "Well, you're Jewish now — what odds?"

15

What odds he experienced the first time he met Grandpa Nathan, a caricature of the gentle, loving patriarch. It was the week in which my husband, Kiva, and I had met in Switzers' basement, having been introduced by a bunch of students. Kiva was blonde, crew-cut, cat-green eyes, golden-skinned, straight from the Canadian sun. I had arranged to meet my grandfather for coffee in Bewley's. I often did and we'd chat for an hour and eat cream cakes. I brought Kiva along and introduced him. Grandpa, may he rest in peace, looked as if he hadn't heard. He wouldn't recognise Kiva, didn't see his outstretched hand. My grandfather had never been known to be rude to anyone, but he wouldn't recognise Kiva. Suddenly, realising what was going on, I blurted: "He's Jewish, grandpa," and Grandpa beamed and held out his hand and said to Kiva: "So, where are your people from? Do I know them?" In a couple of days, everybody in the family knew I had a nice boy, an exceptionally nice boy.

Kiva was only three years older than myself, but experienced. He'd had affairs he could talk about without boasting, he was outspoken and assured the way Irish teen-agers may be now, but were not then. He was one of a flow of Canadian and American medical students who came to study medicine in Ireland in the 'fifties, necessary rejects from their own educational system which gave preference to returned veterans. That strangers clash and fuse, even temporarily, I never doubt since that experience. The electrifying, *infected* feeling of falling headlong in love happens to some people once, maybe twice in diluted form. I can hardly believe that it happens to everyone, to all the people I know who got married. *Wham,* then for so long afterwards the feeling that there is one being with two bodies, two heads, but quite inseparable. Is that the "one flesh" described in the Scriptures? Can it be achieved to order, manipulated?

Suddenly, I had this complete, jelled feeling as if, without knowing it, I had been in bits all over the place before. Suddenly, I felt part of the world around me, identified with flowers and dogs and birds and sky, knew what it was

the Lord had toiled over during those six days. A total
consciousness of being alive is the strongest memory I have
of that time. The excitement, the weak knees, the flutters,
the glow that shone back at me from my mirror were all
things I was to experience again, but that first time of my
falling in love was the time of my arriving in context as a
human being. It was as if I had been floating out in space
and then ... I arrived, I was here. My world became full of
relatives, all close to me, but Kiva was all of them. He was
my father, my grandfather, my mother, my brothers, my
sister and everyone who had ever given me anything in life,
all rolled into one person. "You feel like a crowd of
people", I told him one day, but the perception was something I could not articulate well enough to share.

I've often wondered, knowing what I know now,
whether *she* would ever have been able to go through all
that — trousseau, engagement ring, white dress, wedding,
the ultimate performance after a life hardly realised,
before a life intended not to be realised as anything other
than a puppet in the script. You fall in love — ah, gotcha!
— the scene is set, props in place, players can't be distracted
from cues, in you go, you're the star turn, the Bride, something old, something new, something borrowed, something
blue and something you. Something you? I suppose I was
niggling her even then, asking questions. And yet, there
was no way she could have been talked out of a wedding, a
wedding in the synagogue, a dress of sixty yards of tulle,
the acceptance performance. By whom and of what?
Tradition. Your father walks up the aisle to give you away.
Give away? But I don't belong to anybody. I'm not a
parcel ... Traditional, makes him feel important, just a
custom. But I don't want to be given to anyone — why
isn't the groom given away? Well, probably because he has
to earn the money to look after you. I see. Advice, most of
it from women's magazines. Countdown to the big day,
finish with dampened cotton wool to set the bridal make-
up and give a glow, now the dress, ah, the moment of
moments, the head-dress, and the culmination of twenty-
seven fittings in the front room of Peggy Manley's dress-

making house on the North Circular road. "You'll lose weight before the day, they all do unless they go the other way," and she dropped some of the pins out of her mouth. Daring Miss Manley would ensure my grand entrance.

A day to remember the rest of my life. Could I ever forget? The big day, blazing pimple on my chin, splitting headache, full menstrual flow. Am I committing a terrible crime against the law going into synagogue, going in like *that?* I think I'm supposed to have told them. Told who? If only they'd let a bride eat on her wedding day. It's like Yom Kippur and I can't manage the skirt of the dress, sixty yards of material. I got the idea from the Victor Sylvester ballroom dancers. It will be just my luck if the skirts upon skirts burst forth in a blaze of crimson glory. I think they have; if I could only look behind. Gloria, is my skirt OK in the back? The child smoothes it: "Of course, it's lovely ..."

Please, may I have some water? Water, water, the bride wants some water. She's not supposed to have water. Better she should faint? Bring water ... That's Auntie Ena, blending tradition with commonsense. The water is like a full meal and they powder my chin and fix my veil and ... "They're ready for the bride." The men, praying, are ready for the bride ... My pimple stings and I lift up my skirt and put on the Liz Taylor expression I've been practising in the mirror. I walk into the synagogue, my hand resting on my father's arm, he looks anxious, a bit distracted. Maybe he doesn't want to give me away after all? Naw, he's just not used to this scene. Towards the Chupah, the canopy is covered with flowers, my Grandpa and Grandma are beneath it to one side with my mother who looks too young to be the mother of the bride, blue-black hair framing her face, eyes wide and blue. In the middle stands the groom, Akiva Akuna * * * , named for the famous Rabbi, his surname taken for the town from which the Russian Army chased his parents. He smiles and I stand beside him in front of the Chief Rabbi and the ring is placed on my index finger and the Rabbi disapproves when I slip Kiva a ring too, taken from the best man. The glass in the blue velvet bag with the gold-embroidered Star of David is placed on the floor. Silence. The groom concentrates, raises his foot, brings it down with all his force. Smash; there is a titter of laughter. No doubt. That glass is smashed forever, like a hymen. Only two have shared it, ever can. Mazeltove, Mazeltov.

"Mazeltove, Missus ..." someone says. My stomach turns over. Why do I feel this fading, fading feeling? I haven't eaten. Nanny used to make such lovely soda bread ...

I'm so steamy, like a melting chocolate truffle buried beneath all those skirts of tulle. All my consciousness is focussed on the awful seepage, my body's betrayal on the one day I'm supposed to be pristine, acceptable, with nothing to hide. All those calculations, and now, whoosh, this bloody nuisance. I'll be able to sit down soon. Stop smiling for the Kiddish. I stand solemn while the wine and food are blessed by the Chief Rabbi. At last people are nibbling and sipping and I slip off to the ladies' room, sure that my unimpeded exit is due to everybody *knowing*, they can smell it. Auntie Zelda is in the ladies', waiting for me, hissing: "Your mother told me your condition. Don't let him touch you until you are clean again. You're supposed to go to the Mikva first, but make him keep his distance anyway." She stopped, maybe interpreting my expression as horror of an unknown fact of life, and then went on: "Well, don't worry, *he* won't, but some men are beasts ..." I'm common property now, I feel, nothing will ever be secret again. The tentacles of the tribe are around me. The claustrophobia I felt at that moment in relation to groups in general, and the cumulative affect of the Jewish community in particular, has never left me.

Where did all those people come from? I never realised my father knew that many people, had that many business connections. It's as if he's showing off, I thought, but showing what? People get married all the time. Ah yes, came the nasty little whisper, but they weren't the daughters of mixed marriages marrying nice Jewish boys going to be doctors. A few friends of mine. None of the groom's; just the best man. Mazeltov, mazeltove, people keep telling my beaming father. Chopped liver, chicken soup, roast chicken, pickled meat, gherkins, potatoes mashed with schmaltz, cuggel; toasts — the groom makes the most romantic speech promising always to treat his bride like a Queen. My aunts smile, overcome. Everyone smiles. Only one aunt grins as she digs for wax in her ear with a hairclip. I'm delighted, looking forward to being a Queen, and try to sit up straight and look worthy, but my back is aching; after the cake and tea comes the dancing. Each time I rise to dance I'm afraid my skirt will prove my disgrace. Each time I return to my chair feeling demeaned, somehow. Why? Such lovely compliments from everybody about my looks, my dress and what a wonderful wife I'll make ... I'm just cranky, but I smile. Miraculously, my skirt remains pure, concealing my disaster, and I dance with my legs aching until at last it is a respectable time to creep away. "What are you leaving so soon for?" hisses an aunt suspiciously, "you can't do anything ..."

I'm on my way out of the ladies' room when I meet my Auntie Marie, fairy godmother of my childhood, smiling, eyes brimming: "Eastie egg fer Junie," she sobs, her plump little figure, amazing hat and three-quarter length gloves making her a dead ringer for England's Queen Mother. The hat is knocked askew as she puts her arms around me and I hang on gratefully to the happiest part of my childhood, the sunlit years of Pembroke Road, its feminine powdery smell rising from Auntie Marie's neck. For seconds I'm free and small and I remember letting go her hand when she showed me the huge Easter egg in the shop window. I'd held out my arms towards it, uttering the phrase she made immortal, and home came the big egg. During the past forty-five years she has never considered for a second whether it might be appropriate to repeat that utterance of my infancy, no matter what the circumstances or who happened to be present, and if she lives to see me buried I know what her epitaph will be. Standing there in the hall with her my body seemed suddenly to calm itself. I felt lighter, even comfortable, and we walked back into the reception together. I probably did look like Liz Taylor when I threw my bouquet of gardenias; "Eastie egg fer Junie" rang in my head and I laughed as I let go the flowers. Home to change and out of the pile of tulle, sitting after me on the floor, a dream come true turned nightmare in my memory. We drive to the Shelbourne Hotel on St. Stephen's Green and I flop down on one of twin beds, wondering as Kiva whispers in the hall with the best man. My husband comes back into the room: "Did you know it's the duty of the best man to show the sheet in the morning, to prove the wedding has been consummated? I told him forget it. Tradition, I suppose. We should have eloped. The waiter's coming up with tea and aspirin. Do you feel any better?"

"Who's he supposed to show it to?" I asked curiously, and we both fell about laughing at the vision of the best man waving our marriage sheet from the hotel window. We stood at the window, holding on to each other in spasms of laughter as we thought of bits of interesting evidence of our future accomplishment which we could offer to Dubliners on their way past St. Stephen's Green in the morning. We had baths and after the tea fell asleep in our respective single beds.

2
BRIDE

I awoke next morning as spotless as a bride and as we drove off to Donegal I kept wondering why my body had betrayed me so on my day of days. Conflict? And yet I couldn't have said about what ... How could I possibly know? The wedding thing with all its ritual and paraphernalia was sanctioned, tradition, unquestioned ... obviously I was the one out of step.

I have to say, in fairness, that I had demanded the tribal wedding. *I* got myself into it. I *had* to get married and it had to be quick and not because I was pregnant, but because that fusion of young lovers brooks no argument. The personal reason was invincible enough, but then there were the rules absorbed. If you fell in love and he asked you to marry him, you should say "No"? Go explain to a fat, poor woman that there is such a thing as too rich or too thin. The knight on the white charger was not mythical after all. My prince had come. Not only that, but he wasn't just one of the kids I'd gone to Zion Schools with. He'd come across land and sea and was tall and handsome and blonde and a nice Jewish boy going to be a doctor. There he was, offering me his all in exchange for ... in exchange for what? I didn't ask. His "all" seemed plenty.

Having got the man, found the other half of myself, I zonked into the ego-trip. He thought of eloping, but I wouldn't take the suggestion seriously. No, I was going to have my day, in those days at least the one ego-trip permitted a girl. Happiness, excitement, radiance, call it what you will, it is the stuff that cloaks the anticipation of the engaged girl's ego-trip in which most women are still snared. Look at me, somebody chose me, wants to marry me! In preparing for the wedding I became a property, a property of my own parcelling, of my family, community, tradition. My prince had come and my identity was going. Still I wanted people to see, to applaud. I watched myself with vague embarrassment, not knowing the reason for such uneasy feelings.

In fact I hated my wedding day, every bloody minute of it. It was like an awful play in which I had centre stage, going from one act to the next, through one song-and-dance routine to another, bruised, confused, bloodied, out of touch with why I was there. The day seemed to go on forever and I was aware that when I left the reception, the curtain still had not fallen. Anyway, I thought in Donegal, it was worth it. Something you have to go through and then it's just the two of you.

On the fourth morning we woke to find the groom's face more recognisable as Charles Laughton in "The Hunchback of Notre Dame". The doctor came and gave pills and called me "Mrs.". I felt that fading feeling again. The distortion got worse, the pain unbearable, and finally we drove back to a Dublin dentist, Kiva dosed with pain-killers. After the dentist, we went to the flat over the grocery shop, waiting for the infection to subside, hiding out from everybody. Inevitably, after we had been married a week, someone spied a light in the window and the whole family trooped in to visit us.

* * *

Looking around me I often wish I was beginning as a young woman now. Youth is no longer being wasted by young women. That so many of them are aware of their potential as people, put such a high value on that potential and are prepared to plan and work and, above all, fight for it, never fails to impress me. My daughter is totally in command of her own life, fully aware of her responsibility in its fulfilment. And yet ambivalence born of newly-found choice and confusing rôle-models must be a stress factor in their lives. I wonder about the private struggles of young marriages trying to take new form in an old shape. The shape hasn't changed. The engagement, the wedding day, the husband, the wife, the home — the home yawning for children even while they both get on with their careers. Then the children arrive. Maybe he's a struggling salesman and she's a fully-fledged doctor, but when the first child arrives who is going to be home-maker?

In the early years of my marriage I wrote a short story about a young mother who goes through her days fantasising that she is a doctor, a journalist, a pilot, a business tycoon. She has two small babies but one day, jolted to reality by a minor domestic disaster, she realises that she doesn't have a stethoscope around her neck, her editor isn't waiting for copy, she's not landing her plane in the Andes and there is no big business deal afoot. She applies for a job, hires a baby-sitter and goes off all dressed up for her interview. She doesn't get the job right away, they'll be in touch, but she is pleased that the boss interviewing her is so warm, even affectionate. He smiles a peculiar smile more than once and she wonders about the smile. She goes home, starts to change out of her interview suit and in the mirror catches sight of the nappy pins she fixed to her lapel when she changed the baby before going out ... It's no harm dreaming, she decides, but how could she possibly think she could escape being a mother?

I wonder how I'd write that story today, and yet the country must be full of women with dreams of self-expression outside their rôle in the family, peeling the spuds, vacuuming the corners. Not that being a mother is any less fulfilling in my mind than it was twenty-five years ago, but nowadays I realise that men can also feed children, wash clothes, scour cookers, do shopping, scrub the loo, make decisions as to what to have for dinner, drop kids off in play-school, pick 'em up again, fill my chest of drawers with clean knickers, bras and tights as surely as I have always done for them. The game's up as far as male chauvinism is concerned and I can't understand how any conscious young woman can rationalise the song-and-dance routine of bygone days. Feed him, dress him, arrange his environment the way he wants it, design his social life, be the sex kitten and the earth mother? You've got to be kidding ... And yet I once did all that and felt embarrassed and grateful that the man I married was not overtly a male chauvinist. He vacuumed, washed dishes, scrubbed floors, changed nappies, without being asked. *I* was relieved; that other one felt embarrassed in front of her friends and grateful to be helped with *her* work.

If I had the doing of it over again, I would marry the same man at that time, have the same children and be divorced again. The happy years, the total love experience was worth the anguish. And yet, I think I could explain myself as I am now to him as he was then. I haven't a clue, though, what he has become. Re-married, probably to a feminist. Two different people, even as I am myself.

* * *

Playing house occupied the first months of our honeymoon existence. It was different from other couples because we could be together day and night for a few months before he had to go to college. Within a month I was pregnant. A surprise, but then I am always surprised at how much of a surprise pregnancy can ever be. How could it happen? How could it be? I'd been instructed by aunt and mother to visit the doctor in Merrion Square to get a diaphragm or Dutch Cap. I knew contraception was illegal among Catholics in Ireland but I didn't realise I was breaking the law when I went to see an eminent gynaecologist. It was only years later, on the Contraceptive Train from Dublin to Belfast, that I realised the full implications of the lack of family planning in Ireland. There was the rhythm method, of course, but nobody seemed to know how it worked. If it did, they certainly didn't offer to tell me, and neither did the consultant. His public patients managed as best they could without his smuggled contraceptives and as best they could might mean as many as twenty children, ten not being at all uncommon. But they were poor women, women of Dublin city in the 'forties and 'fifties; I had four guineas.

The waiting room in Merrion Square was full of magazines and two very swollen women ahead of me. The magazine on the top of the pile was called *Brides* and, looking forward to my wedding, thumbing through the frothy pages of clothes, cakes, receptions, flowers and interior decorations, it seemed to me that the purpose for which I had come was less than bridal; sordid, I might have said, had the word come to mind. Eventually the two swollen women were gone, the waiting-room felt enormous with a punitive capacity of its own. What it could do to me I was not sure, but as I sat I became so afraid of it that I made to get out and almost had my hand on the door when the starched nurse opened it and said: "Dr. God will see you now."

He saw me alright. It was the first time anyone had ever seen me in such a way and to this day I wonder what kind of a mind thought up the gynaecological chair. I can think of no worse torture than simply to be left propped up in those stirrups, my backside bare, my eyes on the ceiling, hearing the normal noises of Merrion Square through the net curtains outside. To complete the torture all you need is a strange man, pretending not to be aware of your discomfort, not to be interested in you as a peachy young woman, standing between your legs, pulling on rubber gloves, parting the lips of your vagina with thumb and index finger, saying "relax" in a soothing voice and then, less patiently, "I can't do this if you won't relax," and then plunging the freezing tongue-like instrument, the devil's own penis, up my insides.

"Ah yes, we can fit you," he said reassuringly, and was there a hint of disappointment in his voice? Why?, I wondered.

"I will never, ever, get into that contraption again," I thought, stunned and amazed by it. Who designed it? What demon thought it up? How did he face people with his invention?

"Now," said Dr. God, "I'm going to show you how to

insert the cap. It is very important that you put this cream on it and you must always put it in before intercourse." Six months before, I wondered? Would it stay put? My face flared; he was standing with one foot on the step of the chair, holding a stirrup with his left hand and in his right was the cap, like a dwarf's transparent plastic skull cap with a rim around it. He squeezed the rim together, the better to slide it in himself, and then asked me to do it. I still had no knickers on. "Put it in the way I did and take it out again." I looked at him haughtily, took the sticky damn thing and proceeded to shove it up, trying to keep my skirt draped over my waist as I went. Amazing room up there.

"I've lost it," I said, mortified and terrified, "It's gone, I've lost it."

"Well, get back up in the chair for a moment, Miss Levine."

I stood there staring at him, paralysed: Hail Mary ... blessed art thou among women. "Are you feeling alright? Do you need a glass of water?" ... and blessed is the fruit ... I'd plunged my hand in, caught my middle finger on the rim and plop, splash! the thing flew across the room.

Cool as cool, he walked to where it landed, picked it up, gunge and all, washed it in the basin, shook it, dried it, patting it in a feminine sort of way in a towel, squeezed more cream on and presented it to me again: "Now once more to make sure you have it right. It must cover that knobby thing hanging down inside, that's the entrance to the womb ..." He handed it over almost cosily now. I took it as carefully as I could, gripping it in the middle, and pleep! off it went towards the door. Silence. He let me retrieve it this time. I handed it to him. He nodded towards the wash-basin. Obediently I washed, shook and dried the nasty little thing and squeezed cream on it, walking towards the step of the chair as I held it carefully between finger and thumb.

"Now," said Dr. God, "If you get it right just once more I won't ask you to do anything nasty to yourself again ..." Ah, so my embarrassment was permissible? I shoved the thing up inside myself, letting go.

"It's fine," I volunteered.

"Let me see." He nodded towards the chair.

"No, I won't, I can't ..." dangerously close to tears.

"Come now, you're going to be a married lady. What's all this foolishness, up you go for a second ..."

Up I went. Men didn't have to go through this, I thought. Not their fault, but still. I'd never make love if I had to do this every time. God!

"Perfect," said Dr. God, "good girl, now take it out and wash it."

The chores completed, knickers forming a barrier between me and my recent experience, I sat opposite him at the desk.

"Now, I'll give you this, but if you know anyone going to England or Belfast tell them to bring one and give it back to me. Size 95. It's the only way I can get them, you know. Don't forget now, leave it in for eight hours after intercourse and that liquid stuff in it when you take it out is normal. Good girl ..." I was out in Merrion Square again, my mind muttering to my childhood Friend: "Mary, aren't women plagued? I don't suppose they had them in your day ... Blessed art thou among women ... aren't we plagued, though?"

I doubt that I ever got the hang of that "thing", hitting some part of the bathroom with it every time it sprang from between my thumb and forefinger. Pregnancy seemed a small risk to take compared with the struggle with "the thing". Since one was always "in the mood", which was how the doctor described the occasion upon which "the thing" should be slipped in place, it meant getting completely out of "the mood" before I had achieved what was to me a difficult feat. Scrambling around the bathroom floor in search of the escapee, fingers sticky and smelly from the cream, at best cooled my ardour, at worst put me in a vicious rage. I never did progress to a purely clinical relationship with the cap, and I believed the story I heard of a girl whose baby was born with the plastic-rimmed thing attached to its head. Nor did

28

I ever get over that awful feeling I had for the first time in that chair, legs astride, caught in stirrups, disconnected from the waist down from the rest of myself. It was a feeling which embodied such a mixture of feelings. Shame, yes, but why? After all he was a doctor and I had to be examined, but then why did I think of that incident when I was eleven with the old man who worked in his back garage across the road? As well as shame there was helplessness and panic and inevitability and yes, rage, but I had no right to be raging at that doctor, had I? Had I? On that occasion and through the years those feelings never failed to flood me, to devastate me, every time I put my feet in the stirrups, offering my arse for inspection, probing, disassociation. And always that incident in the shed would return to play itself like a movie through my tortured mind.

He was a white-haired man, thin and probably Protestant because of his grand accent, neat garage with all the tools in place on shelves along the walls. He had a cup of tea on the table in a nice flowered tea-cup. I hadn't realised he lived on the opposite side of the street from us. We were all, a bunch of us, running around and had gone up the wide back alley. We chatted to the man who was carving his bit of wood. The others went off with themselves, but as always I was fascinated by woodwork. My father's craft, cabinet-making; it had often occurred to me as a small child that if I were a boy I'd make things with wood. To this day the smell of sawdust grips me with nostalgia and brings my father to mind — hair dusty, work-coat sawdust coloured, his fingers stroking a plank and making an unspoken decision about what the texture told him. The old man in the shed was carving, the shavings falling about his feet, and an animal was emerging from the block of wood.

I stood beside him, wearing a pale blue dress with little pockets over budding breasts.

"That's a nice blue dress," he said.

"Yes," I said, "it has pockets. We have visitors coming so I hope I don't get it dirty ..."

"Mmmm, nice little pockets," he said, putting his finger into one and moving it back and forth, making me feel funny. I wanted to move away, but couldn't, and he put his finger in the other pocket: "Nice little pocket," he said and I felt very strange and was afraid he would know it.

"It's not every little girl would let me put my fingers in her pockets," said the old man, "nice little pockets ..."

"Harry?" called a female voice, "it's ready now, Harry ..."

"Come back to-morrow," whispered the old man and as I turned and ran, the half-formed animal lay on the table in its trap of wood. I never went up that alley again, but dreamed often about that animal in the block of wood, trying to get out, unable to move, and the voice as I lay on gynaecological chairs with men diving into my insides: "It's not every little girl would let me put my hands in her pockets."

It wasn't until fairly recently when I joined the Dublin Rape Crisis Centre that I realised how much my feelings, on my back, up in stirrups, had to do with the rape experience. "Not every little girl ..." he'd said and how was I to know whether that was true or not? My shame and my guilt bound me to silence, so that not even my mother had the chance to proclaim our sisterhood and declare him a dirty old bastard.

And not even the last time I was in a gynaecological chair, a woman between my legs on this occasion, did I have the courage to say: "I experience this as rapacious. I can't cope with it." There were no stirrups, though, in Dublin's Well Woman Centre and Dr. Máire Woods, a founding sister of the women's movement, just chided: "Ah, come on, June, open your knees, pretend I'm looking down your throat." And I did, but why did I gag? I gagged in spite of her natural manner, her lack of pseudo-detachment or caricatured professionalism, in spite of her warmth and sisterly amusement at my coy behaviour. And then I went home and told Meg who helps me in the house a few hours every week: "I'm jacked, feel as if I've done a day's work and all I did was go to a nice woman doctor whom I know and have an examination."

"The kettle's on," said Meg, "It's those bloody students each havin' a poke, isn't it? You feel as if you aren't a woman at all, just something to be poked at. Put you off sex forever. Not, mind, that I know what all the fuss is about in the first place."

I didn't tell Meg that there were no bloody students at the Well Woman Centre. I didn't have the heart. Class isolated us from each other. Meg had never had a private examination in her life. For each of her eight children, she'd gone into a big maternity hospital as a public patient. A crowd had examined her the first time she ever went — "They talk about your parts and all as if you were an ol' car or something" — and for most of her children there had been students there to "help".

"You think they're finished with you," said Meg, "and then somebody, maybe one of those foreign fellows, asks a question and you're told: 'Stay there, mother,' and there you are with your backside in the air until he knows his lessons. Still, I suppose it's the only way they can learn ... I always feel frightened, though, as if something awful is going to happen. I can't explain what it is. I suppose I do be embarrassed, like."

* * *

We were going to be parents. Ah well, we'd manage. I could do freelance journalism at home, he could find a part-time job. I started to vomit. All day, every day, and eventually in the delivery room of a Dublin nursing home on Easter Monday. Why, I raged as I bent over the lavatory or puked off the platform of the bus, was there such a sneaky conspiracy among women? Traitors. Why didn't they warn me how bad it was going to be, the opposite of glowing and flowering, crawling around half-dead month after month, exhausted, bedraggled, nauseated; you couldn't trust women. They were glad when you were landed in the same trap as themselves:

"You knew and you didn't tell me ..."

"Would it have made any difference? Anyway, some people are never better than when they are pregnant."

"Holy Mary ..." why didn't they tell me about the *Pain*, the tearing, explosive, world-filling *pain?* Delivered of a baby boy in less than an hour, pain, pain ... natural childbirth my arse, grateful for the mask on my face, waking up to vomit and seeing the nurse carrying a swaddled baby across the room. Must be mine because of the pain ...

"How do I know he's mine?"

"Do you think we have babies left all round the place? A baby apiece for each mother, if you're lucky. But sure don't you remember him being born? We only put you out for the afterbirth."

"I wish somebody told me about the shaving and the pain."

"You'd have to be shaved. You couldn't have a baby with a lot of ol' dirty hair. Are you a bit cranky? A cup of tea soon and then a rest. Pain is it? Sure there's a woman in the room above in labour since yesterday morning. You had no pain at all, mother. That poor creature upstairs, now ..."

The poor creature I'd brought into the world was only four and a half pounds in weight and was unable to hold down any meal, including my milk, for the first five months of his life. He could hit a wall two yards away with a spout of milk, no bother, and what the doctors knew about the condition was nil. Concerned and kindly, they told me to do this, that and t'other. His parents obeyed every order, quarrelled over whose turn it was to get up for him at night — both wanting to do it. Eventually my mother, wise old grandmother of thirty-six years, suggested we try him on a bit of porridge. He sucked the gruel off the spoon, it sticking no doubt to his ribs in a way milk could not, and was soon ready for ritual circumcision.

Naturally, as a woman, I was not allowed to attend my son's circumcision. I baked and cooked for the crowd of men who would attend this event and "snack" and drink his blessing afterwards, and I stayed in the bedroom with the women while the deed was done. I hated the whole business. As the years have slipped by I have become more and more in touch with the nonsense of ritual. Step on a crack, you break your mother's back. Nick off that sliver of skin from the infant penis and free him to walk proudly in the footsteps of his unforeskinned forefathers. Ah, but he had forebears who weren't Jews, didn't even have penises. I didn't speak of it. I whispered the Psalm of David in my mind and was in the middle of the Hail Mary when I had a brilliant idea. I got a tiny bit of sponge cake off the flan made by my Auntie Zelda, wrapped it in a bit of cheesecloth, twisted it into a ball, dunked it with whiskey and offered it to the sacrificial infant. He lapped it up. I took it away, he roared. I dunked it again and he sucked happily: "You can't do that," said one of the aunts, "They won't do him if they realise he's been drugged. It's like an anaesthetic. They might decide to come back another day. You can smell his breath."

The child slept. The godparents came, placed him on a velvet pillow, and carried him into the men. I could hear chanting. I was in a rage. The women looked puzzled. Then there was a baby's shriek, though brief. I buried my face in my hands. More chanting, happy sound of male voices, congratulatory sounds. The door opened and the godfather handed Adam to me: "He's done," he said, "He belched in the Mohil's face. He stinks of whiskey," he grinned. And later we had a hung-over baby and a tiny thing to be re-bandaged every time we changed the nappy.

I never remember feeling alone during those early years of my marriage. And I was aware that other women of my age were quite alone. Their husbands went off to work, they stayed home, their jobs were clearly defined. I had married a pre-med student. He tried to get jobs but in the early fifties there weren't many, certainly not part-time ones for foreign students. He had a lot of time and preferred to spend it at home, so a lot of the chores we did together. He could wash and clean and vacuum as well as I could, certainly with less effort. We didn't talk about the fact that he did these things, he just did. I felt myself fortunate that he could take care of things while I wrote an article or went uptown. I remember Kiva was polishing the hall floor in his underpants one day — to save his trousers

— when the door-bell rang. I panicked. I pressed him to get up and get dressed quickly and open the door and meanwhile I'd pretend I'd been doing the floor. He was amazed: "Surely it's only Marie and Manne and they've seen underpants before."

"Men don't polish floors," I hissed between my teeth, "get up." He didn't and they saw he had been polishing the floor and I felt mortified.

Every night at six my father called in on the way home to see the baby being bathed. He and Kiva would fuss over the child in the bath until he was ready for bed and then Daddy would go home to his tea beaming all over his face. My mother would have been with me during the day or we'd all have been round with her. And with one child there didn't seem any good reason not to have a second. What difference? So with two children our lives were completely tied into a family unit, with extensions all over the place, seeming to treat the whole thing as if it had never happened before. As the years wore on, and, happily, the children got bigger, I began to find the whole family entanglement claustrophobic.

"Is this all there is going to be?" I asked myself secretly, never saying it out loud, feeling vaguely trapped. And yet hadn't I all the baby-sitters I could want, relatives prepared to fight for their turn at baby-sitting, a fantastic husband (everybody said so, after all), a son and a daughter and masses of friends? Students from the Royal College of Surgeons came to visit all the time and talked about their interesting studies and travels and plans. Then they all came together at least once a week and were so approving of me, paid my baking such compliments, showed me their exam papers.

There were women among them, some students, some wives of students. I remember feeling confused by the American wives. They all had university educations, they didn't bother much with make-up, they talked about politics and world events, they were looking forward to their husbands graduating so that they could return home and work and help their husbands to their feet and then have families. I was a bit in awe of them, their plans being so set, but found it still puzzling that they had gone to college and intended only to use their education for a short while. Why bother with all that? It was, of course, the era of "togetherness" being talked of so much in America, and perhaps this is why I cannot remember any of the couples as individuals — just a unit or a double human splodge, depending.

Domesticity is only unbearable to most women when it excludes them from the world, from the lives of their husbands and from social contact. To this day I would return to that early experience of domesticity in my life. To have one's living and working under the same roof, to share the things that are done for the benefit of both, is the basis of equality between men and women — but, more than that, it prevents the divisiveness which drives the sexes into separate worlds. It is this sense of "being in the same place" which separates the rural experience from the urban one. Perhaps farmers' wives don't have it quite as good as I did in those early years, but they certainly don't have the same sense of isolation likely to assail your housing estate wife alone all day with domesticity, vaguely aware that what's out there is the important thing, feeling that nature intended women to wash the Y-fronts of the world.

We didn't know it then, but what he had was freedom, freedom made possible by financial and work conditions which did not make life itself of secondary importance. Kiva shared the nappy washing with me, I shared his study with him. Amazingly, there came a day when he brought home an exam paper and I could answer more of the questions than over half of his class. If I'd been a boy, I thought proudly, I could have been a doctor.

The goal, the mutual goal, was his graduation. When he was a doctor all our dreams would come true. We could go back to Canada, the land of milk and plenty, sunshine and snow, he'd get a job in a small town, make a lot of money and move into the city. This was roughly the plan of most of the Canadian and American doctors then. As the years dwindled down, I became anxious to leave Ireland, to make a fresh start, to be free of the intense involvement of an extended family existence, to have some money, to travel.

Then the day came when we were to graduate. Kiva walked up in his gown and mortar-board to accept his degree. Why do I always see him thus in my mind's eye, walking along towards the platform, realising our great moment? Then there was a big going-away party, everyone congratulating me on being a doctor's wife, and we left for Canada the following week. We went on the "Empress of Australia", an emigrant ship of the 'fifties. People stood on the docks singing their relatives off, the air thick with that tearing sensation of separation, the Irish contingent well-sauced, ourselves then unaware of the times that were in it. Unaware of the forced exit of people who had no hope of work at home, no knowledge of when they might be back, not much desire to go in the first place.

It is one thing to long to be free of family "crowding", to desire in one's twenties the chance to establish one's personal boundaries, to cut loose. It is quite a different matter to accomplish this without cutting off one's nose to spite one's face. Suddenly, in my bunk aboard the rocking "Empress", I was aware of myself as an orphan, sisterless, brotherless, and my country, my beloved damned country, behind me for, God knows, forever more. I woke my children up to cuddle them and felt hostility towards this stranger who had come and carried me across the sea. It was as if nothing had happened in between — not our marriage, our years together, our plan to return to his homeland — just as if I was carried off by an invader. I didn't voice my feelings, simply wept myself into a state of exhaustion, and the next day it was all put down to sea-sickness and leaving home.

3
MRS DOCTOR

I had promised to write to everybody, but wrote as little as possible. I never seemed to know what to say about Canada and my life there. Yes, it was beautiful, yes, there were great opportunities, yes, we were well ... Our first stint in St. Boniface, the twin city with Winnipeg in Manitoba, brought our third and last child and was my first experience of what Fay Weldon describes in her book *Down Among The Women.* Our apartment block was in the hospital grounds and now Kiva was gone all day or sometimes all night. The flat consisted of a kitchen, a bedroom, a bathroom and we slept in the living room. My mother-in-law lived in Winnipeg, a woman who had walked across Russia pursued by Army and police, got to Canada and believed it was the promised land. She was the personification of the matriarch, tough, managing, generous. To boot, she was more puritanical than the Puritans themselves, of whom there are a goodly number in Canada. I didn't realise all that then, just that she was a typical "mother-in-law"; the total opposite of my Irish mother. She was aghast at the improvidence of our having three children, but had such a hang-up about having children at all that she would speak to strange pregnant women at the bus stop, saying something like: "So, you need to have a child? Can you afford it? You don't think there's enough children in the world?" That was merely a quirk, but I came to understand that her real fault was simply that of trying to be perfect. She so nearly succeeded that it made her impossible.

She and her brother (who had also gone to Canada from Kiev) were the last survivors of a family of thirteen children who had been raped to death or otherwise killed by successive armies of Russians. Her mouth, twisted to one side in her old age, lives in my memory as a caricature of pain. She simply didn't trust the world at all, and had no time for frivolity unless it was programmed, as, for instance, her weekly games of Canasta or her matinee trip to the cinema. She believed in abortion at a time when I thought it was merely a dirty word and she told me she had done everything she could to try to abort Kiva, her youngest son, who arrived during her change of life.

"You mean," I blurted out, fired by my Irish perception of such an action, "that Kiva, my husband, could have been an abortion?" The family roared with laughter. My father-in-law, a quiet, invisible sort of man, beloved by all, remarked: "But it's true, Brushka, he might not have been here ..."

"So I'd have missed a lot of struggle and worry and slavery and thinking whether we'd have what to eat for the child. A bad thing?" she demanded, looking at the son she now treated as a Messiah.

She knew what every item cost in every supermarket within two miles of her home and was aghast that I hadn't a clue about prices. Her cooking was remarkable, taking hours to accomplish transparent strudel pastry, gefilte fish packed back into the fish skin, cake and biscuit boxes always full. Her house was so clean that before she visited my sister-in-law for the first time, the couple went around their home pretending where they would look for dust or dirt if they were "Ma", and thereby detected every faint offensive speck. And we, her daughters-in-law and her daughter, tried to win her favour, to please her, to give her pleasure, by doing things "right" for her to see. It came easier to the others. I never quite got ahead of the posse.

My mother-in-law was quite well-educated in Russian. She put a great store in education, a value common among Jews, especially those who have experienced pogroms. I recall the visit of a Professor of Literature to the Sabbath meal at my mother-in-law's house. All through the meal, for which she had cooked up a storm, the educated ones at the table — her children thus by virtue of her agonised scrimping to find college fees — talked of great authors and poets, inevitably coming around to the Russians. Trying to draw his gracious hostess into the conversation, the professor asked: "Are you familiar at all with Anton Pavlovitch Chekhov, Mrs. Berns?" She looked up, her Russian accent intensified by embarrassment, and confessed: "Only in Russian, Professor."

Why did I permit her to become my rôle-model? She was so different from the women with whom I had grown up. And yet she wasn't all that different from the young women who lived in the apartment block with me, the other doctors' wives. One of them was a doctor herself, with one child and one expected, and when I met her on our many trips to the laundry room in the basement I hid my unbleached tea towels from her. She carried her stack of laundry in her basket as if it had already been ironed. Their floors were cleaner than any floors I remembered in Ireland, their cooking fancier, their involvement in the means of living more intense than their involvement in life itself.

They were devoted mothers out in the snow playing with their youngsters, they spent afternoons doing what couldn't be done while small children were awake, they knitted, sewed, made curtains and cushion covers. The corridors smelled of fresh baking. A lot of them had degrees, most a good education, but they had found fulfilment in days spent as Dick's wife and Bill's mother. I had arrived in Canada at a time when housewifery was at a premium. And for the first time I started meeting women who saw psychiatrists, took pills, had problems. Lisa had to leave the apartment block and go into hospital. I saw them carry her out one day when I was making my terrified way across the ice to pick up the children in nursery-school. Her husband told me later that Lisa had difficulty in accepting her rôle. Kiva nodded, I offered another piece of apple tart. I didn't know what on earth he was talking about. My family had never used words like "rôle". I couldn't let myself down with my ignorance, so when he left I asked, "What's wrong with Lisa?"

"She doesn't like being a wife and mother. She doesn't want to have this child and she can't stand house-work."

"Why did she get married?", I asked, sisterhood a thing of the future. "What can she do about it now?" He smiled approvingly at me. I gave the house an extra polish-up the next day.

They gave Lisa a lot of pills and shock treatment after the baby was born, and then she went home to her mother in Detroit and eventually got a divorce. She had the two kids to rear and I heard she got a job and predictably re-married. I don't know what she did about her "rôle". I was an avid magazine reader in those days, mostly I think because I had neither the time nor the concentration to read books. Two magazines in particular I had read since my early marriage, *Woman* and *Woman's Own*. Kiva referred to them as my "weekly rubbish" and delivered them with a bar of chocolate, whereupon I was all set for the night. They were like trade magazines, they reflected my interests, my work problems, my aspirations. Of course I wanted to know how to hold onto a husband, prepare a barbecue, clean a room, organise a countdown for Christmas dinner, paint on the right face for the right year, look fantastic on a next-to-nothing clothes budget, give a room a new look with a few cushions. Of course I wanted to be a perfect woman.

I read every scrap of those magazines, and obeyed a lot of the advice. I worked harder than if I'd had a taskmaster, and when we went to live in Saskatchewan and I got a job on the *Regina Leader Post* because money was such a problem, I worked even harder proving that as a working wife I was not unfeminine. Nothing was being neglected because I worked, my appearance was not suffering. I had quite a work rhythm going between home and office, still boning up on my trade magazines when we moved to Arkona in Ontario. There were no papers there, not even a library, but seven churches for the 200 souls in a lovely village in the Ontarion fruit belt.

The doctor's house was big and old and rambling, in need of repair, and sat on an acre of unfenced land, lush with trees, peony rose bushes, and hundreds of bulbs hiding out until springtime. There hadn't been any doctor there for two years or more and the local Lions Club had found my husband. They helped him to buy the house while assuring him that patients would pour in from a radius of twenty miles; I didn't see it until the day we arrived with our children to move in. It was old, rickety, shabby it's true, but what possibilities, what potential to show my magical powers as a homemaker! A bit of paint here, a touch there — I had plenty of work ahead of me. The Lions Club were so glad to have got hold of us that they provided a loan to keep us going until the patients started paying their bills, and offered us a warm and royal welcome. We were vital to the town's existence, befriended and respected by everyone.

Everything would be great, I was told. The country was a great place in which to bring up kids. I'd never spent much time in the country, and wasn't that keen on the outdoor life. Looking back I realise that the shoes I wore, my mummifying clothes, my hair-styles and image taken from the pages of a magazine, had no place in the country. I couldn't tramp over fields or scramble about the country dressed in my "natural" gear. Neither could I entertain the thought of letting myself go — into flat shoes, jeans and wind-blown hair-styles. To-day, I would love Arkona — for a visit. It reminds me a bit of County Wicklow, and nowadays I am glad to be in the countryside when the weather is not hell-bent on rejecting me. But I'm Dublin born and bred and appreciate the things a city offers, anonymity, work opportunities, newspapers, crowds, traffic, shops, theatres, cinemas, restaurants, parks, easy access to friends, the lights down O'Connell Street, fish and chip shops and the smell of the vinegary bags in people's hands, the last bus home, the emptying of the pubs every night, the first editions of the papers on the streets. To be close to the Mail Boat Pier, as the crow flies from Georgian Dublin, or within a bus-ride of the vitality of the Liberties, is my security.

Twenty years ago I hated the country, its loneliness, its strangeness, its inconvenience, nature's indifference. So that day when we drove into Arkona my heart sank. Countryside all round, green and lush, and in the main street, such as it was, women in trousers and sneakers. Not a picture house, not a hotel, not a pub ... And then, later, in the community hall, I was introduced to people as "Mrs. Doctor" and learned that I would be taking over the surgery. Everyone wanted me to know how wonderful Clara, the last doctor's wife, had been and since I was, after all, the doctor's wife, I proceeded to act out the script awaiting me. It occurs to me now, of course, that had I questions for which answers had not, as yet, been voiced. Never during those years in Arkona did I escape being "Mrs. Doctor". The Lions Club had got themselves two for the price of one and I didn't even notice that I wasn't offered a salary. The doctor sat in his surgery; his nurse, the "Mrs. Doctor", received and assisted him and ran the home through the dispensary wall by remote control.

Anyone who says housewifery is not competitive ought to read some books about the American housewife of the 'sixties, or experience what I did in Arkona. The doctor's wife had to be "best" at everything, and her kids had to be cleaner, better-mannered, brighter in school. Whatever about being, like Caesar's wife, above suspicion, certainly the doctor himself was God and the conflicting vibes I picked up from other women in the village had a lot to do with their fantasies of being married to a man who was The Doctor. All the time I kept up with the magazines, visited the hairdresser's (forty miles away by car), took up gardening and won prizes for my blooms, took up bottling and freezing as if a famine were imminent, and prided myself on having the linen out on the line before nine o'clock of a summer's morning. I disappeared into the enormity of the house, refurbishing, keeping it going, never satisfied with my own efforts.

My day went something like this: up at 7.30 a.m., get the kids washed and dressed, breakfast, answer telephone calls. Get the youngest organised or prepared to follow me around while I cleaned the three-room surgery and loo. The first room caught all the snow and mud from the overshoes in the winter, and smelled like a pig-pen in summer. Clean down the front steps, dangerous to the patients when icy. Now into the surgery — all the time answering the phone, taking messages — clean the mess left by polyps, abscesses, bandages. Empty dirty containers, sterilise instruments, re-cover the examining couch and polish its stirrups. Shine floors with the lovely machine I got for my birthday, on into the back room, dust and polish, freshen up loo. Time for a cup of tea, race upstairs to groom "Mrs. Doctor". By now it would be 10 a.m. and I cleaned half of the rest of the house while answering phones before lunch. Lunch, and eventually the doctor would arrive back from the hospital, whistling importantly, and walk past the kitchen saying: "I'll have something later, there are people waiting out front." No lunch, so I put the youngest down for his nap, finished cleaning as much more of the house as I could, did some ironing or gardening or preserving, made afternoon tea, delivered it to the doctor, started getting the dinner. At night I usually ironed, baked, did some more house maintenance, gave myself a face-pack from the recipes in *Woman's Own*, did the washing and held it over for hanging out before breakfast.

By this time, contraception had become a problem of the past. The pill arrived in the dispensary office; I was given some samples and continued taking it for ten years. If it caused depression, increased appetite, loss of libido or fluid retention, it was all in my imagination, my husband said. It had been tried and truly tested and could not be the cause of anything. So I took the pill. It is also true that sometimes I helped myself to samples of slimming pills in the surgery, on the quiet, of course; the temptation was too much. I weighed five pounds more than I had when I married and I had never been the right shape anyway. I started having my hair lightened; it was too black. No matter what I did with myself, though, I was always wrong. My clothes never looked as the magazines promised they would, my skin was never as fine as my care should have made it, I didn't walk properly, my legs were too short, my boobs too big. It was all desperately frantic. The house wasn't the way I wanted it to be either. It took so much to keep up. Even when we could afford help, I expanded the amount of work to use the hands available. When we got a nurse in the surgery, there was still so much to do I was always exhausted. One Yom Kippur, we went into the synagogue in London, Ontario, and met some couples with whom we became friendly. Their wives were perfectly groomed, lived in perfectly appointed houses with picture-windows, had finished their work by 10.30 in the morning, had Canasta games three times a week, cooked fantastic food, gave dinner parties and had everything in the dishwasher before we waved them goodbye and went back to Arkona.

They were all college-educated and I felt a bit inferior, but they were friendly, busy, happy and gave no inkling of discord within themselves. I joined their voluntary groups, such as The National Council of Jewish Women which sprayed charity in many directions, towards the plight of the American Indian, towards long-term mental patients trying to make it back into the world again, towards study projects. They awarded me a pin for my work on behalf of human rights — speeches mostly about the condition of the Red Indians. Something started to happen in my head. It was as if some little cog went into motion and disturbed the rest of the machine. I wanted to learn about things, to have some education, to be able to join in conversations wherein were dropped the names of writers, poets, scientists, politicians, names other than my beloved Shaw, O'Casey and O'Connor. I didn't dare care about a degree, since I'd left off my formal education in primary school, but I wanted the knowledge.

They didn't want to take me in the University of London, Ontario, at first, but when I explained that I would pay the fees and work hard if they just let me sit in on the degree course and mark my papers and I wouldn't expect credit for it, they agreed. I got first class honours and didn't have a clue about what I was reading — not consciously, anyway. The struggles of the people of the new world for freedom and independence struck a nerve but did not turn me to my own need to find my feet, my own thrust towards growth. "Imagine," I remarked one day, "Tom Paine saw women as enslaved ..."

And yet, slowly, inevitably, something had started to change in me which was distant and indefinable, but relentless. I couldn't name my malaise, nor could I rationalise having it. Everything was the way it was supposed to be. The house was now easier to run, redecorated in most parts; we had daily help. My husband was successful, wonderful, my children were fine. I drove a lovely new car the forty miles to London to the University and to shop. I was expensively dressed, my hair was perfect. Some of my most unhappy hours were spent at the hairdressers, sitting there helplessly being styled, wanting to have it look just right, full of irritation, something like a scream in my throat.

I couldn't name my problem. I would disappear into moods of dank despair, slither down slimy walls of darkness, to emerge again slowly, exhaustedly and raging. My sex life had become dreary, but I had dutifully learned to feign orgasm and convinced myself that really these things were not important to women. That "these things" had once worked very well for me I rationalised as natural to the honeymoon period. Besides, how much energy did either of us have left over at the end of the day?

And among the women, the Arkona women, one smiled the "Mrs. Doctor" smile and in London one was the happy "Jewish Mamma" playing Canasta, doing good works. My rages, like my despair, seemed to have no basis at all. It was the era of togetherness, with "his" and "her" towels; friends even had double-seated Elsans in their country cottages. The magazines said you had to communicate; one or two couples had "little problems" they discussed with marriage counsellors, working on true togetherness. I insisted on talk sessions. I carped and carped because I couldn't put words on what was really wrong; he interpreted, the doctor, always knowing best: I needed an afternoon nap, a holiday, a trip back to Ireland, a better sex life, more clothes. We wouldn't always be in Arkona; there were better things ahead. Talk, talk, talk.

I would wake up in the morning, the sun shining through the gossamer gold of the curtains, and groan: "Oh God, not another day," and then take a tranquilliser to get me through it. Why was I so weary? And being weary why couldn't I simply rest, recover? All that was expected of me was to be a normal, natural female. Why couldn't I do that much? I would be tending my flowers or doing something around the house when suddenly, as if all the stuffing had gone out of me, I would stop, sigh from the roots of my being and say aloud: "Is this all there is ever going to be?" What was my problem? What did I want, for Christ's sake?

While I was disappearing into "normality", seeing my perfect image reflected in the gleaming floors of femininity, sniffing appreciatively the odourless air of spotless bathrooms, dazzled by my whites, Betty Friedan had been writing her *Feminine Mystique*, the ultimate description of the "problem that has no name." The cover of the book spoke of America going back on the emancipation of women, the deep malaise which gnawed at the happiness of so many American housewives, caged in comfortable homes, loyally conforming to the pretty, fluffy image of the magazines, but condemned for life to a spiritual death and continually asking "Who Am I?"

I wish I could say that book changed my life. It could have done, perhaps it should have done. It did not. I remember saying: "Yes, that's me, that's how I feel ... but." The "but" was to be my downfall.

What could a Mrs. Doctor, zonked on tranqs, miles from the nearest newspaper, with an education vastly inferior to her new-found peers, do about Ms. Friedan's observations? Besides, I doubt if I took in much of the book at all. I used to skip pages of books then, found it hard to concentrate, and perversely had an impatience with women who were intellectual and different and outside my own reality. Yet having lost most of my material possessions of those days — even my precious collection of china cups — how do I still have that copy of Friedan's book? It's yellowed, and I discover marked in shaky ink: "American women lately have been living much longer than men — walking through their left-over lives like living dead women. Perhaps men may live longer in America when women carry more of the burden of the battle with the world, instead of being a burden themselves. I think their wasted energy will continue to be destructive to their husbands, to their children, and to themselves until it is used in their own battle with the world ... And when women do not need to live through their husbands and children, men will not fear the love and strength of women, nor need another's weakness to prove their own masculinity. They can finally see each other as they are. And this may be the next step in human evolution."

"Who knows what women can be when they are finally free to become themselves?", asks Friedan. Certainly, I didn't have a clue to the answer. I remember trying to read the book, struggling with its dense, studiously weighty learnedness, wondering what my mother in Ireland would think of it and deciding she wouldn't read it if I sent it to her. *The Feminine Mystique* increased my confusion, irritation and depression, or was it that those conditions made it impossible for me to grasp the book's message, its validation of the female condition, its raft-like offering to those who could recognise the possibility of a light at the end of our tunnel of domesticity? I thought I was like the women Friedan wrote about, but felt that we had made our beds and must lie on them. Women paid for falling in love, having children, paid for lovers growing into husbands, women paid, paid. Water flows down, not up; men have penises, not wombs. Nature didn't have to be fair, she was the boss. She? Yes, I remember the hopeless realisation that I'd made my bed and if the lumps in it were hurling me into the pits, so? I couldn't make it again. Best I could do was to adjust, count my blessings.

Then, too, Friedan was a different kind of woman, a woman I dismissed as being outside the pale in those days. I could bet what she looked like, masculine, plain, feet planted in walking shoes. After all, what *real* woman could write a book like that, could have all those resources? How could she really know what life was like for a girl like me? I was twenty-nine years old and had three children, and still did not call myself a woman. I'd always been married to a man, though. It was only much later that I realised that Friedan too had had her share of feeding, washing, shopping, only later that I realised that our sex had turned us into a profession, the profession whose work it is to let the other half of the world get on with their lives without having to be bothered with the details of creature comforts. Our profession made it possible for most men, perhaps not all, to answer the vital question early in life: "What do you want to be?"

Of course there was the problem, for me, of culture, of language. American jargon confused me, seemed unreal. What would people at home think of "rôle", "identity", "self-actualization", "fulfilment"? I could hear the jeering Irish laughter even at that distance. Strangely, I did not truly believe that my nameless problem was the same as the nameless problem of all those other women. Anyway, by now I had gone past quiet desperation. I was into intense pain. If there was a solution I could not imagine it, could not shape it in my mind.

Compared to my mother's life, mine was a cake-walk. Dare I look for a solution to a cake-walk? But then, in 1963, the year of the first edition of that book, I was burrowing towards that unique solution to things — madness. "Madness" was a taboo word. I was depressed, anxious, threatening to have a nervous breakdown, unstable, call it what you will. I call it madness. To me madness is a place, a terrible agonised place where so many of us go and are totally alone. Hell is not like madness because hell is not an escape from heaven. Madness is an escape from other people's sanity. And no matter what they do to you when you are mad in an effort to make you like themselves again, you fox them anyway because madness is a place of one's very own. In there you feel what you feel, cannot feel what you are supposed to feel, think what you think, dare to be yourself. They make tentative steps to get in to coax you out, drug you, treat you, try to cure you, but you stay there until it might be safe to venture out again. Who else, save Nature, could create such a place as madness?

4
MADNESS

I did not head for Madness in a straight line, nor could I direct anyone there, having been. It is, of that I am sure, a place within oneself of which everyone is aware at some level at least some of the time. We know the place, surer than hell. The people who make it to Madness get there by strictly individual routes. Some arrive slowly, inevitably, some shoot like a rocket out of disaster. You can't be driven there; it is a journey which needs total involvement. Other people, their expectations of you, circumstances, may create the need for the trip; the going is of one's own volition.

A lot of people mess about between sanity and madness for all of their lives, neither shitting or getting off the pot, passing on the constipation of emotion as a legacy. I lived for a cruelly long time without breaking completely. Nowadays you could say I was in a stressed state, but "stress" as a description of feeling had not become popular then. What it felt like was an on-again off-again state of pain with an underlying awareness of life. And as time went on, the pain deepened when it was there, all the feelings sharpened, becoming monstrous caricatures of themselves. Despair, terror, irritation, anger, distrust — the feelings kept for occasional experience became everyday expressions for me. When I was afraid, it seemed as if I was only fear, a fear which could touch others and make them fearful, for I could see it in their eyes. Everything would, I remember, get inevitably worse before menstruation and then lift afterwards as if a black three-day rainfall had ceased and light was released. Now, battered, relieved, I would struggle upwards. Eventually, though, my relief at the lift of pain and crushing depression carried me up until I became "too happy", unsuitably high.

I never did anything terribly drastic in those moods, I realise now. After all, it was the time when the Kinsey Report was being written and Americans were discovering that a surprising number of nice suburban wives like me were having affairs, that they were breaking out of their perfect moulds into jagged patterns of bewildering delinquency. Looking around me in my high moods I was simply enthusiastic about doing what all the "normal" women around me did all the time. I filled my time with shopping for "perfect" outfits, children's clothes, household things. It took me two weeks, six hours a day, to find sheer drapery material the golden colour of an autumn leaf I had pressed in the pages of Yeats. Then for days and days I sewed them — I who cannot put a button in place now without bunching up the material — covering the huge bay of the bedroom with them to create a glow as of the leaves outside smouldering mellow. And within the room was the mood and dignity of an old country place of my dreams, with warm wood, a golden crocheted bedspread, a rocking chair and stool in which a New England Puritan might have needle-worked her life away.

God, the shopping that went into that house, into my life then. Perhaps the only freedom greater than having one's own money is to have someone to spend it for you, spend it to titillate your taste. To say, perhaps, "I'd fancy a room like that," throwing across the magazine, and have the little woman run off and attempt it on the money available, ah, there's the power of money, plus. Then there were all the hair-styles, hours spent lightening hair too dark, straightening hair too curly. Cooking, bottling, freezing, stocking up. Going to the beach and maintaining a tan. Important to be tanned. Important the shade of the tan. Scraping pubic hair away from the bikini line. Christ, the itch. Toffee apples, for Halloween, red and lusciously sticky on popsicle sticks for every child in the village; lazy to give a handful of sweets, especially for the Mrs. Doctor.

What was it Snow White's dwarfs sang? "Busy doing nuthin', working the whole day through, trying to find lots of things not to do ..." I filled my time with work that didn't count as work. Why was I so exhausted, so tired? Might as well take a tranq, nothing special about today. In good weather, though, always the beach, and my toddler son Mike. "Speedy Gonzales" played hourly on the car radio, and he drummed it out incessantly with his spade on the sand bucket. Best company in the world, pre-school Mike. "We don't havta eat samidges just 'cos we brought them," he said one day, "we can buy hot dogs or even nuthin' and throw the samidges in the trash can ..."

Freedom? Just a word for not eating samidges just 'cos you brought them.

Suddenly, maybe after a night out or in the middle of some gay activity, this awful hollow feeling would fill my insides. Emptiness. What's it all about? Is this really all there is? Now I knew I was on my way down, down the thickly slimed walls, down under weight, under darkness, down where tasteless food, odourless blossoms, mimed sexuality and children without magic formed a vacuum of joylessness in a world which otherwise appeared to go its own sweet way. It was while I was in the hollow state, the state which would eventually lead to rage as I fought to defend myself against the descent into the pit, that I first went to a psychiatrist. It was an order. Either I went or we got a divorce. It never occurred to me to ask; what if we got a divorce? I had never, coming from Ireland, heard the word divorce spoken seriously, and its effect was amazing. An explosion went off inside my throat. That's where most of the pain was, always, in my throat; my head seemed to fill as if with something solid like cement and my body became a sort of passenger. Inside the head, so tightly packed, the word "divorce" kept repeating itself. Divorce, divorce, divorce, but meanwhile I smiled and smiled and moved obediently in the direction of the shrink.

I hadn't had an ordinary doctor for years, partly because there wasn't one we could easily get to, partly because somehow, along the way, perhaps during the years when all those medical student friends of ours were becoming doctors, I had lost respect for the profession. I remember well, for instance, my shock at a party when I heard one doctor say to another: "Go back for the appendix on another trip. Another fee, man." And yet I had known good doctors, medics with the vocation, the healing touch, back in Ireland. In my childhood there had been a Dr. O'Leary on South Circular road who used to bring his patients eggs from his farm, and on his way out of the house when he had delivered my brother Norman in the night, he was singing: "... I'll fix up your troubles and go on my way, any umberellas, umberellas to mend to-day?" Perhaps familiarity bred contempt? In any case, for years my husband had treated all of us for every-day things. My daughter once, aged about seven, said: "Daddy, please, I'm too sick for samples, get me some real medicine from the drug store."

So Daddy picked a shrink for Mammy and told him all about me, and one night we drove the forty miles into London and I met the man who was chosen to make me feel what was expected of me. I was not, I was told later by my husband, in a very glamorous condition the night I met the shrink. I had this old black beaver coat into which I burrowed, the fur comforting the palm of my hand as I gripped it closer in front. My black hair straggled greasily around its collar, my face was ashen white, a streak of lipstick drawn like respectability across it. Apparently my nails were chipped, and my appearance totally unacceptable for the purpose of having my head examined. I remember these details because I have blocked out all other memory of that first meeting. Weeks later my husband told me how I looked. He was trying to make me realise how ill I had been, I suppose; he also mentioned how embarrassed he had felt meeting his colleague with me in that condition. I was seared with shame. I've never felt so ashamed of myself since. Had I really let myself go like that? I knew that the female crime, the uniquely female crime, of letting oneself go, was the pits. Had the handsome shrink made his first impressions of me in that state? My mind floated back to Dublin and a forgotten incident of those days.

It was a Dublin day, one of those sopping wet days when Americans always seem so well equipped with macs, umbrellas, plastic things for their heads and rubber things over their shoes, but we Irish, being particularly bloody-minded about our weather, squelch around complaining about the wet, refusing to prepare for it in the slightest, refusing even to refuse to prepare for it. Kiva had stayed home to mind the baby. Bubbula, that was what he called me, "little doll", had set off wearing a grey flannel hobble skirt and jacket and black stiletto shoes, with a very large silky print scarf of grey and red. Off I went, with the faith of the Irish, into a morning patch of sunshine. The Irish attitude to the weather is similar to our attitude to birth control: Ah, sure, take a chance. Naturally, it rained buckets all day.

On this morning, I ended up five miles away in Moore Street, buying fruit and vegetables from the women on the stalls, women without macs or umbrellas. By the time I had made my way back to the bus for home, stopping for a cup of coffee and a bit of a dry out in Bewley's, I looked exactly like a typical Dublin woman on a wet day. I had been drenched and dried out a couple of times before I finally made it to the bus 200 yards away from the house. Brown paper bags were bursting, stockings spattered with mud, hair tight to my head like black candyfloss, silk scarf so wet that I cheerfully wrung it out in the sink while the kettle boiled.

"Who saw you like that?" asked the blondeness of my life, his voice heavy with dismay. "Do you know what you look like? To think of my wife being seen like that ..." Oh God, I thought, I've broken every rule in *Woman's Own* and for weeks afterwards I trod daintily about the place like an elegant visitor. I had not yet used the expression "fuck off", nor could I, then, have understood its political implications. But I remembered that day years later in Canada when I found myself once again in the dock. This was not even my *first* offence, I contemplated morbidly. I'd done it again. That day in Dublin, and now worse. Worse because this time it was in the presence of an Important Man, a man who could tell things at a glance, a man who could judge how mad and bad I was, a man who could glance at me and *know*. I still don't know to this day what it was, if anything, he knew because I don't think he ever told me and if he did, I've forgotten. I remember once he asked me if I had a goal, if any one thing I could think of would make everything OK. I couldn't answer him. What did he mean? Wasn't I a married woman with me markets made, as they said in Dublin? So I told him about my husband's goals.

The shrink was about forty years old, quiet and calm and pipe-smoking, kindly, with a habit of flushing and studying the smoke from his pipe very closely. I started dressing up to go and visit him. In fact, my visits took on the atmosphere of dates. Getting ready was like those times before the hops in Dublin's rugby clubs. You had to have something different to wear every time. I found him extremely attractive, everything I thought my husband had been, and for a time my arrival in Madness was delayed by the sustenance of this fantasy relationship with my shrink. My wardrobe grew rapidly, my appearance improved, so did my mood; again I'd found someone who understood me. That is what those grunts from behind the pipe meant, I'm sure. I had, of course, developed transference. Of course I hadn't a clue, and thought I'd fallen for my doctor.

I was obsessed with him. And of course the obsession made me guilty. I couldn't talk about it to my husband because I was afraid of making him jealous. Besides that, he might speak about my "crush" to the doctor and I'd have died. Just died. Nobody bothered to tell me that transference is a part of psychiatric treatment, a good thing if handled properly. Transference, I now know, is simply the shifting by the patient of the most relevant feelings in her life on to the therapist. So I had transference. I won't attempt to say what the shrink had. It is always better to let professionals name their own feelings, since they are always right and the rest of us are so easily confused by these things. Besides, I was unstable at the time. Quite unstable. Anyway, the psychiatrist and I got along fine as a pair, except, of course, the problems of my life were not being solved.

Things went on like that for quite a while. I had spent an odd week or so in hospital having a "rest". Then an unexpected thing happened. I was driving back from London to Arkona one afternoon. I'd left the hospital, all dolled up as usual, and went into a London car park to pick up my car. There was a bunch of young men getting into another car. They said something among themselves; I knew it was about me. My back felt cold, but I trotted up to my car saying, "Good afternoon" primly, as I slipped behind the wheel.

"Yeh, sure," said the dark one putting a bottle to his mouth. They all stared. I backed the car out in confusion. Why was I so upset? I drove out of town and had still not shaken off the feeling when I noticed that a car behind seemed to be going to pass. It didn't signal, but drew closer and closer. It was the men from the car park. They were making signs at me to pull over to the shoulder. I knew I must not. Now they connected with my back bumper, shunting me along. A bottle flew out of their window, rolling into the ditch ahead of me. We were fifteen miles outside London, with twenty-five to go to Arkona. "Have a drink, lady." shouted the one who had said: "Yeh, sure."

I sped ahead as fast as I dared, leaving them behind. They raced after me until their bumpers connected again. I put my foot down now, sweating, terrified by the feel of the floor, no one to scream to, not a soul on the road. With my right hand holding the wheel, I emptied my handbag onto the seat beside me. Fifty-six dollars. I threw the bill-fold out the window. They were close again now. An ugly hoot of laughter: "Hey, fellas, she's trying to buy us off. How about that?" I sped on, my foot down again, now sick with the fear through which all men keep all women in subjugation. The new Dodge would not go any faster, but they had let go of me again. Cat and mouse. They intended to keep this up; already they had developed refinements of the game. Now, when they were within a yard of me, they would stop dead and give me a head start. I'd rolled up all the windows, was looking desperately for some kind of weapon. Against a car full of them? Oh my God, if there was only something to crash the car into. I might only roll over in the ditch, make myself more vulnerable, the black car upturned like a beetle. I could feel my bowels loosen; blood dropped from my nose into the pale pinkness of my lap. I had started praying my way out of this world when suddenly a miracle, a miracle disguised as quite an ordinary thing, happened. A car appeared on its way out of Arkona, five miles away. And then another one came along, a neighbour who beeped at me. I slowed down, the car behind followed normally. Into the town, turn left before our corner house and right again and into the barn used as a garage. Now the white car drove past the front of our house, someone's thumb on the horn, until it disappeared into silence some distance away. The game was over. I sat in shit and blood and sweat. Just sat and sat. Then I noticed it was dark. God, why had I worn that dress, those shoes. I shouldn't have spoken to them in the car park. My fault. Things like that didn't happen to other women. How had I got involved with four men in a car? I went into the house and the baby-sitter looked up, startled: "I didn't hear you drive up. Gosh, what happened your dress?"

"Just a nose-bleed," I said. He was out late that night. I asked the girl not to mention about the blood to save the doctor worrying. Had a bath, put all the clothes in a bag in the cellar. Went back to the bathroom to get the shoes. It all had something to do with those shoes ... Eventually, told the psychiatrist: "Yes, but nothing actually happened, did it?"

Years later, when I was doing a training course for coun-sellors at the Dublin Rape Crisis Centre, we were all talking about rape and its effect on women, and about our feelings, when suddenly I remembered that fear in my car that afternoon. It had been a fear like no other, yet familiar, sickeningly recognisable, making other fears trivial. It had a life of its own. It dwelled as a race memory, poised in the pit of my stomach, prepared to grow in relation to one signal, the ancient atmosphere of rape. The opposite of the Sleeping Beauty ... I became silent in the group. Memories flooded in: "Not every little girl would let me put my finger in her pockets ... psychiatrist or divorce ... up you get in the chair ... yeah, sure, ... live better electrically." I was back in the electric shock treatment room in Canada when Ann O'Donnell, administrator of the centre, said: "Hey, June?"

"Sorry," I replied and we went on to discuss why raped women so often think of themselves as the guilty ones. Those shoes ...

That is my last memory of driving home to Arkona, although it must have been a while before we moved into London. By now my husband had become fascinated by my condition and its handling and decided he would take up psychiatry. So we moved again, this time to facilitate his studying in London. And it was about now I arrived in Madness. This time it couldn't be covered up or described as a little rest. The doctor's wife was over the top, she had to be taken into the psychiatric ward. I was to learn pretty fast that while ordinary nurses played along with my "little rests", their nursing fell far short of the reality of my condition. One nurse on the general ward occasionally baby-talked to me. I was glad to leave that kind of insult behind.

It was, of course, a rather fancy psychiatric ward. People paid their way with voluntary health payments. The place was physically attractive, bright; everybody was kind, cheerful and reassuring. The emphasis was on normality. We were all behaving quite normally under the circumstances. Nothing awful was happening. Everyone was doing fine. Well, almost everyone. But there was something in the air most of the time, a sense of the staff knowing something unbeknownst to you, the patient. Meanwhile, if you mentioned that to a nurse, back at the ranch (the shrink's office) it would be called paranoia. That pumping was discreetly done for information and carried to the doctor was beside the point. The fact that you sussed their inter-communication system indicated paranoia. Personally, I had it bad. I made friends with a few of the nurses, flattered to be treated as an equal. Then their little postal system dawned on me.

"Did you tell Dr. So-and-so what I said about ..." I would ask.

"Of course not," came back the answer. So how come the man behind the pipe suddenly knew things he hadn't known?

When you felt well enough to walk around you met other people starting to feel well enough to walk around. The women all seemed to be of the same age, well-groomed, well-dressed. In the morning, if you weren't scheduled for shock or insulin treatment you could knit or paint or read. Then there were the visitors who behaved as if they weren't uncomfortable visiting a psychiatric patient.

My room was on a corner with lots of windows looking out on space and trees. The screens were on the inside though, locked. The door had no lock on it. It had a handle that didn't turn and a window in case it had to be turned into a locked door after all. So the door which could not be closed was always slightly ajar unless you propped it with something and that was against the rules. Nobody said so, but whenever I attempted to close it by putting a wastepaper basket behind it, a nurse would come along and make a great display of putting the basket back where it belonged. Then she'd forget to close the door after her.

The staff could be extremely decent and helpful, but being mad doesn't make you stupid, and I felt insulted by their scant measure of my awareness. They were trained to help the shrink help you get better. So it was rather a once-removed relationship with the nurses when you got the hang of things. Doors that wouldn't close, windows that wouldn't open, friendly nurses helping the doctor to help you. Ah yes, well. The girl next door had a door that wouldn't open, no clothes on herself or the bed ...

Trust. You have to learn to trust people, I was told. Have to let people help you.

"I hear you've been using pretty rough language," said my trustworthy friend, the doctor. "Your husband says you never used to do that. You have never used four-letter words to me, have you?"

I shook my head, intent on shaping a four-letter word. It wouldn't come.

"What are you trying to say?"

"A four-letter word."

"Go ahead, be my guest." Puff on the pipe.

"Help," I whispered.

He looked as if he might cry.

I felt, at the time, like a peeled grape, so vulnerable that I dared not exist and yet with deep feelings of violence. When I wasn't drugged my feelings were of utter distrust of everyone, dependence on everybody. I hung on to my friends, phoned them ten times a day when I could. Still, I felt abandoned, trapped. Eventually, when all these feelings sank under thick depression, I would cry and cry with this terrible sense of loss. Then it was time for more shock treatment. After the shock treatment, the feeling was of confused relief. Within the confusion I was released from a terrible burden of guilt. Guilt and separation seemed to go after the shock treatment. Guilt about what? Separation from what? It was as if I had done something terrible, had to carry the knowledge alone and then at last I was found out and punished. My debt was paid. I felt OK for a while.

We tried to make fun of the "treatment". There was an advertising slogan in Canada at the time: "Live Better Electrically." One day a bunch of us, in the guise of occupational therapy, painted a big sign and stuck it to the door of the treatment room: "Live Better Electrically."

As an out-patient I drove forty miles there and back to

get shock treatment. That means I never saw the carriers because they didn't have to carry me into the room, just out to the resting-room still unconscious. This morning, the "ghouls", as I'd heard a patient refer to them, turned up to take me from my bed for treatment. I was already dozy from something they'd given me. There were four "ghouls", middle-aged plain-looking men in green coats. As a group they resembled a bockety bit of mobile furniture. Between the four of them they had a spatter of afflictions which included a short leg, a twisted arm, an eye patch and a twitch. They may have been war veterans, maybe they were just naturally disabled. They never spoke to me. I think one member of the group was actually un-maimed; he was fair-haired and almost bald. They put me into a carrier thing and brought me down the hall to the treat-ment room, discussing some matters of masculine impor-tance from the daily paper. As I drew nearer that room my prayers to Mary emptied other thoughts. She would stand at the foot of my cross and I was capable of what seemed, then, a bizarre thought; would they crucify a woman spread-eagled? I imagined I could see her, slight figure in a cotton gown and veil, and she had now my mother's face, now my sister's. The door closed and they were left wait-ing in the hall, opposite. Minutes for them, eternity for me. Then there was the vaseline on my temples, the needle in my arm and the awful descending feeling as if one's whole self were sinking into the mouth gag, teeth together, dissolving, blending gum into gum and then that distance of no breadth began to make a whirring sound, whirring, whirring as my eyes opened to the scream of an ice-cream pain in my left eye. I'd arrived out of the mouth gag. Now I was in a cot, looking out through the bars at other cots crowded into a large room. From the cots came groaning, moaning and snoring. The whimper was from me. My God, the headache. Reassuring voices advised sleep now and I slept, not asking if the voice had meant me. Nor did I think of the degradation suffered in the few seconds of awareness in that room with the cots or the "ghouls" who had carried me there until I was forced to go back again. Each time, waking up in that cot was unbearable humiliation. I didn't complain about it for the simple reason that I knew my views would not be respected. The worst part of mental illness is the loss of autonomy. Other people are always right, rational in every way, by virtue of the fact that you are receiving psychiatric treatment.

Eventually, numbed, my memory shattered, the treatment began to "work". I was said to be in better form. Certainly, the rawness, the guilt and the panic were gone. But who was this person walking round? I tried to get in touch with her, sometimes stared at her in the mirror. She was me alright, but she felt unknown to me. Perhaps I was supposed to have been like this all along? Detached, calm, far away from myself, pleasantly smiling. People seemed pleased with me; the doctor, the nurses and the visitors came more often and there were more of them. To appear in truly better form and to impress the fan club, all we women knew a trick that was taken as a sign of health; war-paint. You could be in tatters, but if you got the make-up on, had the hair styled, you were seen to be trying to pull yourself together. Full marks. So we women played girl games, and talked girl talk. We were smiled upon. Encouraged. One nurse would always let you know if the shrink was on his way to see you unexpectedly. Now you scrambled to get on the make-up, spray the room with scent before he arrived. Now he could see that you were living better, electrically.

I had been home for the week-end, home with my husband and children in the new house in the suburban estate. It looked strange to me. I could not remember furnishing it. I had though, and spent far too much money, I was told. Again autumnal colours, a gold-coloured fur couch, gleaming wood floors with throw rugs, Danish furniture. Gleaming kitchen except for the thing on my plate at the table. A lump of flesh bleeding into the pattern of flowers, a potato soaked pink.

"Why won't you even eat?"

I weighed about seven stone now, but sat there, throat tight, unable to stuff the food down.

"It's because she hates blood," said one of the children. "Give her ice-cream. You like ice-cream, don't you, Mum?"

No, if she wouldn't eat her dinner, she wasn't having ice-cream. What had happened to my kind loving man? He seemed spiteful. Impossible. The June before this October my sister Barbara had come to visit me in London and gone home to report: "I think he is trying to drive her mad. He's not the same fellow we knew. He seemed to want to provoke her and she took it. They have this beautiful kitchen with formica counters and he was cutting bread and she asked him to use the board. He deliberately sawed into the formica. I'd have stuck the knife in him myself." A bit sickly herself at the time, she had not pretended to notice anything. "Come home for a bit?" she asked before she left and I felt as if a raft had tossed away leaving me fighting the sea. Then again in the hospital, between treatment, her letter: "Come, come somehow ..."

Now I was glad to get back to the hospital and its bloodless food. The week-end had left me shaking, waking up in the morning feeling terrified, clinging to the sheet. Pills and tea and some sleep and a visit from my friendly nurse ... We chatted. How had my week-end gone? How were the children? Had I noticed anything unusual? Then quietly, ever so quietly, she said: "Look, things can't be OK between you. It can't be all you. While you are lying here, your husband is having an affair with my best friend."

Suddenly, everything made sense and nothing did. I took the sedative offered, which didn't work. After she left I simply lay there ruminating, thinking, "she's made it up," knowing that she had not. I got out of bed, went to the phone and said: "So-and-so says that you are having an affair with her friend, the theatre nurse."

"Oh nonsense, she's just an older woman, years older than me. Nothing like that ..."

So, she did actually exist. Older woman, "just", the ultimate sexual dismissal. I was too overcome with rage to think about that. I went back to my room, through the door that couldn't be locked, and pushed the heavy bureau up behind it. Never physically terribly robust, I nonetheless

63

moved every scrap of furniture including the bed so that it barricaded the door. Then I climbed into the bed and just lay there in a fury. I had to keep them out. I had to lock that door.

"Piss off," I yelled when someone knocked politely, "I'm not letting anyone in here." But they got in, a bunch of them. I was forced to face reality.

Reality, when you are consumed with jealousy, is even more difficult to face. It became like a *dybbuk* in my personality. I was possessed by jealousy. I remember the first time I saw "The Incredible Hulk" on television I identified my demon jealousy with his amazing chemical change from a person to a raging monster. As I watched the character expand into a powerful destructive monster, shirt bursting, skin turning green, I thought: "That's like me in Canada!" I wanted to tear the world down around me with rage. I must have used up most of the jealousy in my system at that stage because I have never been able to sustain the feeling of jealousy for long since recovering from that bout. Of course, my values have changed. Nobody *belongs* to me anymore, not even my children. I'm nobody's baby. I have come to loathe human ownership as a transaction of slavery. I do not claim to be unhurt by rejection, but it is the reasons for one's rejection one fears, the inadequacies in oneself of which one is well aware that form the basis of jealousy.

Jealousy is not about loss, it's about fearing been proven not as "worthy" as the winner. On that basis, how can reason support jealousy? If a lover is discovered to prefer someone else, wants to be elsewhere, what's to argue? Soreness heals, sadness is absorbed, the hollowness of loss fills up. Jealousy exists in its own right, feeds on dependency and insecurity. "He's got all his own teeth, hasn't he?", a jealously raging ex-lover of mine of latter years asked: "that's it, isn't it?" So teeth were my friend's ego-reflection of rejection. Can't you just imagine the poor bugger gnashing his gums?

My own jealousy was described as pathological. I think they meant out of proportion. True, a lot of it was unexpressed from childhood. Stored away like a time-bomb. It had to do with my father's adoration of my sister Barbara, born when I was eight years old. I remember challenging him on this once and he replied:

"Ah, don't be silly, she's only a baby." Just an older woman.

Feelings were not examined when I was growing up, they were patted down, so I never dealt with the jealousy I felt, simply walked away from it as soon as I could. Walked away from my father's house. The confusion, the bewilderment I felt at the time my marriage broke up seemed out of context, even to me. It was the bewilderment and confusion of a child replaced in its parent's affection.

It seemed to me that in suffering a change of heart, my husband had suffered a personality change. I suggested this to the doctor who felt: "No, every personality trait has its opposite in the individual. It's just the other side of the coin, that's all." He seemed to be in a monstrous rage all the time, denying his affair with the nurse until the doctor pointed out that lies were making it impossible for me to sort anything out. So now he decided to leave the house, with me leaving the hospital to look after the children. It was just as well. Every time we met ended in a bitter row, my tongue honed by the agony of it all. Even when he came home on Christmas Day he left in a rage.

With him a student again and with the cost of moving and with my illness, money was scarce. I weighed 90 pounds and was asked wasn't it time I stood on my own feet. So, with three children, I got a job in a department store. I nearly burst a bloodvessel trying to master their cash, billing and exchange system, but managed to be passed by the instructor, who put me on the fashion floor. Why did I choose to work in a shop? Did I *choose?* Well, there was the ad. in the paper and I answered it. In those days I thought that working in a department store was easy. You were just there, helpful, selling things, taking the money. The only thing I would have considered required less ability was housework. *That* did not occur to me. My goodness, a doctor's wife? Anyway, I was so physically below par that I couldn't have coped with housework, not even with the aid of all those machines in Canadian homes. Besides, I knew about shopping, didn't I? Well, not much, it's true. Not compared to other Canadian housewives, who seemed to know the price of every supermarket item within five miles of their homes, but I could learn.

Obviously, my self-worth was blown. I felt bombed. If anyone had told me I had skills, had accomplished anything, ever, I'd have thought they were trying to brighten my day. If I had thought of marching into a newsroom or an editor's office and asking for work I'd have been the first to sneer at my own fantasy. No, if this was a new life, I was on the lowest rung of the ladder, a failure in marriage, in ability to survive, in anything you care to mention. Washed up at thirty-one. Indeed, I didn't even see this new life as a beginning. This was the end, my frozen destiny, and in an early-morning panic I would think: "Oh God, what's going to happen to us all? How will it ever end?" The most likely end I imagined was my own suicide, but then what of the children? I should have thought of them before getting into this mess. The only happy end I could imagine was to wake up from this nightmare. Even now, more than seventeen years later, I wake up with a start the odd time, sick with panic, back in the nightmare. Then I remember: I am no longer a refugee from my husband's life. I'm nobody's baby now. My own person. The limitations of my life are my own doing.

That I passed Simpson's training course and got a job had a lot to do with the fact that they desperately needed staff coming up to Christmas. And yet, maybe that instructor, a crisp, efficient woman in her forties, squeezed me through. The class were in awe of her, but I remember her whispering to me as I struggled with some complexity of the store's money system: "Don't rush at it. Relax. Customers are human, y'know, they'll be fairly patient ..." And another day she asked me: "Were you always so thin?"

I needed the job for the money, but I wasn't able for it.

Sometimes I would go to the ladies' room, just so I could sit. My change of life-style couldn't have come at a worse time. The new student life was proving "exciting" for my husband, now living in residence at the hospital. It was pretty basic for me. I had no car since we could now only afford one. Or rather, he could now only afford one. I had a job that took me downtown each day at 8.30 a.m., having got the children to school. There was a goodly walk through snow, ice and wind from the bus to the house, plus two jobs instead of one. My social life as a single, rather fractured unit was non-existent, as was recreation of any kind. As soon as the dishes were done at night, I was into bed, minutes after the children. I woke around 5.30 a.m., took a pill and felt reasonably pain-free by 7.30 a.m.

I wasn't very good at my job. I was too distracted. The most I could manage was to be pleasant and helpful to customers. In fact, I'd have enjoyed the work if I could have got the hang of things. And the nightmare of every day was the tots, totting up what you'd sold, charged, exchanged, getting out at the end of the day. In this, I was always the last, always in trouble, delaying everybody. The other women helped me, anxious to get out of the store at closing time. They did so mostly with irritability and amazement at my dim-wittedness.

The Christmas shopping rush proved to be too much for me. I simply collapsed on the job one day and had to be taken home. At home was my daughter, Diane, ten years old. Anything she could manage she did without being asked, was forever stroking me and bringing me cups of instant coffee. What was happening since the last day at the hospital seemed to be happening to the pair of us.

When I could I tried to separate from her, be the mother, return her to her childhood, but it didn't work. Our rôles merged; each female served as mother and daughter to the other, depending upon the circumstances. Between us, we looked after the boys, one older than she, the other younger, and if this made them feel excluded, I knew no better to do for them at the time.

It was about this time that Heather Klein came into my

life. Actually, I'd known Heather from a group of volunteer women with whom I'd worked before my illness, and I often wondered afterwards if Heather was chosen by the group for the task of giving me support for as long as I needed it. She hadn't known my husband socially, only me. "Programmed" friend or not, Heather took on the commitment with a heart and a half. Here was sisterhood. A family woman, she was never too tired to listen, never unsupportive, always ready with carefully considered commonsense advice. No judgements. She still lives in London, Ontario, a cultured English woman, loving the arts, gently independent. She fetched and carried me to and from anywhere I had to go, brought cooked dishes to the house, had us for Sabbath meals, took us to the synagogue. Heather had a rare, rare quality, the ability to help without imposing on the recipient. No matter what she had to do for me, no matter what we discussed or what crisis came up — and there seemed to be at least one a day — she protected my boundary as a person. Her attitude was a constant reminder to me that I was a human being with a mind and emotions of my own. I was not expected to do as she might do in any given situation. I was June and she reminded me, always, to be June, not Heather. If, on occasion, I might say to her: "Janna says I should do so and so," or "Evelyn thinks it would be a good idea if I ..." she was almost bound to reply: "What do *you* think? How do *you* feel about that?" I remember once relating a bit of advice given to me by Thelma, a perfect wife and mother. The advice was that I should always look fantastic, hair done, dressed to the nines, scented, in case my husband dropped in which, she warned me, could be any time. On such an occasion I should behave "sweetly and in a lady-like fashion" so that I would make him sorry he had left. "Oh God," said Heather, "I think I'm going to be sick." I wondered what she meant. She was forever, gently, reminding me that it was my life no matter what its current condition. Who could say what was best for me? Obsessively troubled, I was hooked on listening to people's solutions to my predicament. Heather didn't offer solutions beyond: "eat a little of this" or "you need an early night."

I was surprised the day I told her I was going back to Ireland to try and get myself together. "Good," she said, "I'm delighted. I'd hoped you would decide to do that." And yet in all our talks, all my agonising over whether I should or should not go back to Ireland for a while, she had never said: "Go." She had listened and asked questions and nodded and said: "Well, let's sleep on it for to-night at any rate." How wise was Heather, how sensitive to my need to gain the slightest sliver of autonomy. I had lost control over so much. I used to go grocery shopping with Heather and she would stand patiently while I decided what to take down off the supermarket shelf. My indecision was torture. Lamb or chicken, canteloupe or water melon? Did I need more sugar? And she just stood beside me as through a haze of drugs I struggled to do what had been second nature to me once. Eventually, I went back to my old habit of making a shopping list. Heather pretended not to notice, as if I'd been doing the sensible thing all along. Diane helped to compile the shopping list. She also helped me to lay out clothes to wear for the next day. If she didn't, it meant an agonised hour trying to make up my mind what to wear and with what.

It wasn't simply the illness, or the shock treatment, or even the sense of earthquake which existed in my psyche where my marriage had been. I'd fallen so deeply into the acceptance of other people making decisions for me that I had surrendered the responsibility for deciding anything for myself. I was not occupying my own space. My husband had decided I should go to a psychiatrist. He had decided which one. My husband had decided to leave while I was in hospital. The doctor decided I should go home to the children. My husband decided I should get a job. In Dublin they were deciding I should come home for a visit. My husband decided he would not let us go unless I signed some papers before I left. He decided I couldn't have a passport unless I agreed to certain conditions. My doctor decided Ireland would do me good, give me a sense of perspective. My husband decided the visit should take the form of a trial separation. My brother Les decided I ought to get rid of my husband and my psychiatrist. My husband decided I should put our furniture in storage and leave the visit open-ended. The doctor decided I should take the children's toys with me. It was decided — who decided that, I wonder — that my son's Barmitzvah should take place in Ireland. It was only a few months off and my in-laws decided that this was a good idea. My husband decided how much money I could live on. My sister-in-law, furious at her brother, decided we should go to Toronto and leave for Ireland from her home. Diane decided we would need new suitcases and some passport photographs. Heather came to Simpsons and spent a terrible afternoon while I tried to choose suitcases and kept breaking down in tears. We got passport pictures. I still have mine. I look aghast, enormous eyes in a tiny face, looking as if they see something terrible.

The bewilderment I felt is unforgettable. There I had been, fairy-tale marriage, dreams come true, the rich life, wonderful husband, lovely children, part of everything. I'd never realised how, quite suddenly, I could be apart from everything, sharing nothing. I hadn't thought about needing rights. Now I had none. I was like a dismissed slave, a no longer welcome pet. Out. I owned what I stood up in. My father sent me tickets to come home. I was plunged into the struggle of maintaining my dependency. What was I entitled to? What was *he* going to give me? I could feel myself being shaken off like dandruff from a collar, and I clung. My struggle towards independence came later. Meanwhile, I was going back to Ireland, an Ireland I had left behind me in the grim 'fifties, an Ireland with which I was out of touch, although I had never fully succeeded in getting in touch with Canada. Still, it was going to be alright. I was going home to my mother and my sister and I would return in the full of my health, to hold my head high again. After all, this was only a trial separation.

5
DUBLIN AGAIN

Why would anyone in the throes of a marriage break-up
return to Ireland? But where else would I have gone? For
years, home had been where my husband chose to live.
Without him I was a displaced person. But Ireland recognised itself as my home. Dublin was asking me to return. I
could stay in the nightmare that Canada had become for
me or I could make a break for it in the hope that the shift
across the ocean would change something. I was aware of
all the letters to-ing and fro-ing about me between relatives
and in-laws. They discussed what should be done with me,
and tried hard not to imply that they didn't wish to be
landed with my disaster. I didn't, even then, blame them
for being weary. I'd handled disintegrated people myself,
tried to help them. It is so very very difficult. Walking on a
broken leg can be managed with spirit, but it is harder
to reach a crushed spirit. It is that lack of core that is so
difficult to deal with. Talk to a person in flitters and she
can only make flitters of what you say. A woman in
flitters, exploded out of a marriage with the debris of two
lives vibrating around her, is an exhausting task. This
woman was incapable of recognising reality, objective
reality. For God's sake, I hadn't yet called myself a
woman. Women were, in those days, sexually past it. You
were a girl as long as people were flattering enough to call
you that.

This desperate sense of disaster was all I had left of a
marriage I had believed to be, albeit subconsciously,

indissoluble. Even my children were not a great comfort to me. The important part of my marriage had been my husband. People who kept reminding me how lucky I was to have the children just made me feel guilty. I didn't feel the remotest gratitude. But I was anxious to get them to safety.

The people in Dublin would rescue the children. They might have doubts about how to cope — some might even enjoy a bit of satisfaction at my failure — but as my mother wrote, "blood is thicker than water ..."

It was an uneasy feeling, coming home in these circumstances. Strange, how clearly I remember that. Every emigrant fantasises about coming back, returning triumphant, a success, laden down with gifts. The remnants of my pride gave me difficulty. How would I face people? I was one of the walking wounded, but as yet had not recognised which battle I had lost. I remembered meeting people from Belsen and Dachau at the end of the war. They had been convalescing in Co. Wicklow en route to the Promised Land. Perhaps this identification was no more than self-pity, anyway, I looked the part, skin and bone, shocked. What stuck in my mind most about those people had not been their physical condition, but their helplessness. Others were deciding what could be done with their lives. Unlike me, they had been grateful for any chance of survival at all.

I had mixed feelings about Canada now. I felt the brave new world had failed me, rejected me. I wanted to wave my Irish passport at the Canadian traffic that day we had gone to buy suitcases. I had retained that part of my identity, refused to surrender it, been unable to do so.

I hadn't been back to Dublin during my eight years in Canada, mainly, I think, because relatives came to visit us. Now, as I started to leave Canada, I began to experience a sense of relief. I come from a child-oriented family. My parents, their Auntie Barbara, their Uncle Norman, would welcome my children back to the fold, fuss over them, reclaim them from all the heart-ache. There was another element in the relief. Distance might make the heart grow

72

fonder, but it made it impossible to keep the war of my marriage active. Fight or flight: not much of a choice.

We left Toronto on a snowy-white, sun-drenched February day. I was not prepared for the shock of greyness when we arrived at Dublin Airport. Would the sun never follow? I wondered. Oh God, the greyness, as if Nature herself was sighing in despair. Everything seemed dirt-coloured, and there was a greyness about the clothes people wore, a greyness in their skins. The patch-work of green fields, fresher than snow, had not prepared me for this first glimpse of Dublin. We waited in the baggage hall of the old Aer Lingus building, able to see my grey relatives, worried and excited-looking, until our cases came. And then, suddenly, as the glass door slid back to release us, the rescue party plunged into action. The children were swooped upon and whisked off as I had known they would be. I drove towards home with my sister Barbara. She was busy pretending I looked great, well, a bit thin. She failed to disguise her relief at having me here and not "over there on her own". The greyness seemed to lift as the adult that is Dublin emerged along the journey.

I hadn't lived in London, Ontario, for very long, but I had become used to its well-heeled immaturity. It struck me now that it was really only one huge suburb. Not that I'd sought its history to claim that it lacked one, but now as I drove up Dorset Street, past Findlater's Church, it seemed to me all so solid, so permanent. In comparison with Dublin, London wasn't really a city at all. Why, Dublin had been long in the tooth while Canada was as yet a mere twinkle in a Puritan eye. Passing through the city centre which I'd stomped as a cub reporter and knew from my childhood I felt a stirring in myself that can only be described as re-rooting. I had not transplanted well. The texture of this place felt more natural to me.

"It looks great," I said to my sister.

"Yeh," she said, "lovely slums."

"Why didn't I come back before now?" I asked.

She sighed: "Maybe you didn't want to be reminded," she said.

Outside the city-centre hotel where I'd gone to my first dress-dance to discover later that the management didn't want Jews in the place, we were stuck in a traffic jam. I was mesmerised by the state of the traffic. It seemed as if everyone drove independently of other cars.

"You have to be brave to drive a car here," I volunteered.

"No chance of dying of boredom at the wheel," said Barbara.

Somebody behind pressed a horn and kept the noise going. My sister opened the door of the car, got out and stared backwards until the noise stopped. Now, she called good-humouredly: "What else did you get for Christmas?" I was delighted by the Irishness of it all. I hadn't realised until then how proper Canadians are.

Eventually, we drove on over the River Liffey, black and stinking, the tide out, and by the time we had passed the Bovril sign high over D'Olier Street and drove around by Trinity College I was getting the weirdest sensations. My lungs seemed to grow inside my body and blow up with air and this air relaxed me, let me float back in my seat. I had a sense of having been reclaimed. I was conscious of being comforted in the lap of the beloved oul' crone that is Dublin City. I snuggled into her dampness and her smells, burrowing home. Old, battered, tattered, falling apart in places, as good as ever in others, furbished hysterically here, there like an ageing beauty, Dublin welcomed me home. Overawed by her great age, I was proud of her triumph over time, her scars, her dignity. Dirt in her pores, time in her bones, she spoke to me. In response I wanted to get out of the car in Harcourt Street to feel her pavements beneath my feet.

As we drove towards Kelly's Corner I had a sudden curiosity to see part of my childhood's Dublin.

"Could we drive up Clanbrassil Street?" I asked.

"But sure that's out of our way, we're going to Church-town," my sister laughed. It had all been a bit before her time, of course, the shopping street which was in the heart of the Jewish ghetto. It was very much a part of being Jewish when I was young, though. That was before second-generation Jewish immigrants managed to climb out among the native middle-classes in Terenure, Rathgar and Rathfarnham. Off they had gone, the first Jews to move away from the South Circular Road, away from where you'd expect to find Jews in Dublin. They were the cream, the first out to the new suburbs, the successful, the comfortable, the timidly swanky. Timid, because who dared to swagger? Who thought to show pride? Everybody had run from somewhere. And they'd looked on the map and seen Ireland, there on the other side of England and said: "They'll never find us there. That's a good place."

"Did you ever see a poor Jew?", they used to say in Dublin and I was puzzled because the people who said it had more than us. Even nowadays, when people start chatting about the lean years of the 'forties and 'fifties, what I have to say is usually glossed over. With a name like Levine, speaks the air, what would you know about poverty?

Not that I liked Clanbrassil Street as a young adult. It had that cloying, incestuous quality that threatens destruction. Don't tell us who you are. We know all about you. We've decided what you are and what you'll be and nothing will change that. The little shops with their dark, mean windows looked like huddled gossips, cannibalising, licking their chops, washing your blood down with the milk of your mother. Slyly intrusive: "Ah, but you don't keep kosher then." Feigned liberalism. Deep shrug, "Well, some young people don't these days and then it's not easy, of course. Not easy, but if you're brought up to it. I couldn't swallow ..." And years later when they got the money they were out at the Mirabeau in Dun Laoghaire, lapping up Sean Kinsella's fat prawns, tearing at his duckling. But in the meantime, eyes everywhere, tongues beating the tribal drums, and the remark out of the side of the mouth. God, how I used to recoil, as a child, from the oul' nosey parker smelling of cooking oil who'd corner me: "So, whose little girl are you? Levine? Philly's daughter?" and someone would come in: "That's Solly's daughter." Looks exchanged, explaining everything. Explaining my

Irish looks.

I remembered the grocer shop where we always went for the Passover bread and all the other things "koshered" for Passover. "How can a packet of sugar be kosher?" my mother used to ask every year, irritated by the prices of the provisions which were special for that time of year. It must have occurred to my mother that the Jewish God was strangely obsessed with matters pertaining to food. I can still see her standing in that shop, waiting for the Passover order, recoiling at the complexity, not to mention the price, of it all.

"Suppose you just couldn't get the money for all this?" she asked my aunt once.

"There's a fund for the destitute," my aunt replied, "they get for Pasach like the rest of us, don't worry."

"I'm not," said my mother.

I screwed up my nose inside at the back of my tongue before I entered that shop. It smelled of pickled herring. There was this huge lidless jar of fish cadavers in a smoke-coloured fluid in which floated black peppers, onions and bay leaves. The woman of the house plunged her hand into the cauldron to get the herrings. She had two odd hands. One was like corned beef.

Outside, on the corner of Lombard Street, were the fish-women, the mongers, delighted to do business with people so peculiar they ate fish every day, not just Friday. It was worth their while coming to "Little Jerusalem" of a morning, to do battle with the Jewish housewives. Around the baby prams with the boards of fish on top swarmed the women, doing serious business. My mother, polite and gentle, was always being robbed, but a more capable housewife could bargain down a penny here or a few fish thrown in there. And for half-a-crown or two bob you could get enough fish to do for days. Plaice fried golden would go under a wire mesh in a safe cold place and be eaten with horseradish and chips. Or there was the orgy of making gefilte fish, a mixture of fishes minced and flavoured, shaped and then fried or boiled. And my mother could make it better than anybody, she that was reared on hot buttered eggs from the Monument Creamery and plump chickens with daintily powdered breasts from Findlaters. Probably because she hadn't tasted it as a child, she missed out the teaspoon of sugar used by central Europeans.

Nowadays, of course, we used hens, not chickens. Fat meaty kosher hens, bled and still warm with life, their fat oozy, their innards filled with golden eggs. And from that creature you could cook a feast. From a good hen, or even not such a good hen, you made the Sabbath meal, by comparison with which Christmas dinner has always fallen a bit flat for me.

"Why do they eat hens when they can buy chickens?" I once heard a teacher in the Jewish National School ask.

"Sshhh" was the reply. The school was run by Christian teachers who, to give them credit, had shown us not a sign of missionary zeal, the while their relatives saved black babies in Africa.

We drove on towards Harold's Cross, out towards Kimmage, where we had lived before moving to the South Circular Road. Past the grotto at Mount Argus. My sister probably didn't even know that little grotto, ablaze with penny candles, lit by me in secret with money saved by walking home from school. Honeybee bars or candles to the Virgin. Forbidden fruit, more precious than the obligations of my companions.

Past the "Sunner", the Sundrive picture house, near where I had lived in Blarney Park. How fervently I'd believed in the adult life of Hollywood. That was what one grew up to, the romance, the glamour; the "Sunner", but only on Saturday, romantic exotic leading women who sang and danced. It never occurred to me it was for their suppers. Maria Montez, Betty Grable, Merle Oberon, Maureen O'Hara, and of course the terribly foreign Carmen Miranda, always matched with Cesar Romero. One knew somehow that romance with anyone else was out for the Brazilian bombshell.

Will I ever forget when Ronald Reagan had his legs cut off in "King's Row?" I hadn't been let go to it and had sneaked in and staggered home after the picture having experienced the first sadistic shock of my life. A doctor could actually cut somebody's legs off if he liked. "Where's the rest of me?" Reagan screamed when he woke up from surgery. It was a terrible shock. But of course, we all knew it would only make his sweetheart all the keener on him, his having no legs. Her father should have thought of that when he did the job.

"Yes, but what happened after we left the picture-house?" my brother Stanley used to ask, loath to come out of the matinee into the glaring light of childhood in Kimmage. What indeed.

Eventually, we arrived in Churchtown to my parents' house, but not the house they had lived in when we left. Central heating, thank God. By the end of the week we had settled. At the end of the second week, the children were enrolled in schools, wearing uniforms for the first time in their lives; my daughter loved it, pointing out at eleven years old that it was a relief not to worry about what to wear for school first thing when one woke up in the morning. Years later, she told me that on that first day off to school at Alexandra College, Earlsfort Terrace, she had got lost and rambled around Stephen's Green in a panic. Finally, she asked someone directions and arrived for school late.

"It was awful," she said, "everybody was so nice to me, but I felt lost, not just lost for school, but totally lost." I would have been at home in bed, clinging to the mattress, trying to get my anxiety enough in check to get up and face the day. And the child was lost. It had been explained to her where to go, she'd been taken to the bus stop, shown where to get off, and she'd done what she could remember, but got lost. There she was in her strange brown clothes, in a strange bus in a strange city going to a strange school, the product of the unexpected strangeness of parents for she knew no one else then in the same plight as herself. Not here and not in Canada. She came home happily enough, though, and always speaks of "Alex" with special fondness:

"They didn't say they knew about me," she says, "but the teachers were kind and sort of specially gentle ..."

The youngest boy settled into my old school on the South Circular Road. The eldest boy went to the High School in Harcourt Street. Adam was a Barmitzvah boy, supposed to make his Barmitzvah in July, and as yet he had had little instruction. We found a teacher and he started his study. The goal became the Barmitzvah. It was to be a family party in my sister's house and in the beginning we all pretended that there was a chance that my husband would return for the biggest day in any Jew's life. The boy studied, the women made out menus and planned outfits, monthly cheques came from Canada (the amount decided upon there), letters came occasionally for the children, nothing for me except maddening references in the children's letters to "your mother".

I still weighed very little, ate very little and started each day with tearing anxiety. The Dublin psychiatrist diagnosed me as an endogenous depressive. This meant simply that depression was natural to my nature. In other words, it was chemical, visited upon me, nothing to do with what had gone on in my life either now or as a child. The cure was to be pills and rest and a moderate life style and "eventually you will get better." Strange to say I didn't, not for years, not until I was convinced by someone, someone who had no connection with medicine at all, that one could choose to be depressed and anxious or one could choose to be in control. It was difficult. It took time, but I set about doing it, weaning myself off the Parstelin, the chemical strait-jacket to which I had become addicted, one day at a time, like an alcoholic. But this was after I'd joined the women's movement in Dublin. After the dawn of consciousness, years after meeting that man in Herbert Park.

I still, when I remember, say a prayer for that old man in Herbert Park, a stranger on a bench whom I met sometime in 1966 or '67. It was a beautiful day and I was working off Baggot Street. I bought a sandwich and an apple and walked to the park. I was sitting there, watching the ducks, as I would have done long ago when I was a child living with my mother's family on Pembroke Road nearby, when this old man on the other end of the bench struck up a conversation with me. He must have been at least seventy years old, and poor. I sat up beside him and we chatted. We talked so long I was late back to work. He told me of his boyhood in Dublin and of his wife's death: "We were more like brother and sister, y'see, we were that close. She's left a big space in the world ..." He'd gone on to talk about her, to tell me all about her, so that to this day I see her in my mind's eye, a black-haired girl from County Clare with huge green eyes and a lithe figure, quick to giggle. She'd come up to Dublin to look after an aunt of hers who was poorly and they'd met.

"And wasn't that the lucky day?" he'd asked me. I was overcome by the old man's memories and as he pulled the cork out of an old medicine bottle to drink his milk I started to cry. And then, of course, I told him about my "nerves" and he was very interested and asked me questions. And when I'd told him my story in the simple way I perceived it in those days, he took my hand between his own and said: "Child, look at me." And when I did, he said: "How do you think you should feel after all that? Depression is it? Pills? Doctors?" His lashless old eyes filled with tears.

"Isn't it that your heart's scalded? Sure, don't I know well? Ah peteen, how would you expect to feel?" I was amazed by what the old man said, so amazed that I forgot to take his name when we parted and although I returned to the park to look for him I never found him.

I've said that to many a woman since: "How would you expect to feel? What's sick about feeling the way you do with your wounds?" Usually, it works the way it worked on me. Suddenly, in the fog, I could begin to recognise a cognitive context of life. Conditioned as a female to blame myself for everything, for not fitting in and doing as I was expected, I began to realise that the world had no right to expect so much of me. My pain was hard-earned. Perhaps there is such a thing as endogenous depression, but in any event, how could I expect to feel? If only I had met that old man in Canada; what a therapist he could have been.

During the first months home in Ireland I did what the doctor told me, took the tablets, I took them every morning with the tea brought to me by my father before he went to work. By ten o'clock the acute anxiety would subside and I could manage, numbly, through the rest of daylight. The months passed in the domestic company of my mother and sister and Marie Berber, a friend from childhood. I seem to remember ironing. Did I spend the afternoons ironing in my mother's kitchen? She could never understand where I found all the clothes to wash. Then the Barmitzvah had passed and I was well enough to want to get on with life. A trial separation? OK. I must go back to Canada, and try to work out my marriage. It couldn't be done from here — not with a man who had always been bad at getting his thoughts down on paper. I'd always written to his relatives for him.

The arrangements were made, the day came to leave and packed bags stood in the hall. We were having our last cup of tea before leaving for the airport when a telegram came: "Do not want you back in Canada. Letter following." I could have continued the plan, of course, but "Do not want you back in Canada"? The women who had been drinking tea simply cried, or looked white and bewildered. The men were silent. The flight was cancelled. We left most of the luggage packed until the "letter following" arrived. Those few days found me in a fugue. I became obsessed with the word "why?"

I'd squint my eyes and stare into space and someone would ask what I was thinking about and I'd say "nothing", and go back to trying to figure why. Why? Why? Why? Why was I being treated like this? Why had I no say in anything? Why had I to wait for a man to ask me to marry him and why could he say "Don't want you back in Canada"? The whys of my childhood tormented me. I was surrounded by contradiction. Men had power, money, strength, wisdom, the deciding word on things. Yet they always seemed to let women down. Why did we depend on them? Why did we trust them? Females seemed to live in a world which centred around a man or men to be pleased. Why? Why was it all so unfair? Why so cruel? Why did women believe that marriage was the ultimate security when clearly its stability and happiness depended on pleasing the man and keeping him pleased? Why hadn't I seen it all before? Why hadn't I realised that marriage, for women, was just another word for slavery? Why couldn't women see the danger? Why hadn't I protected myself against this savagery? Why had I accepted slavery? Why did the women, so sorry for me, not realise that they, too, were simply slaves, even though slaves in good omen? They were proud to be in good omen, proud not to have been cast out, like me. Proud to have done *what* right? Why? And the most awful why of all — why had I not realised all that power was there before it was too late? Why couldn't I have been the way I was supposed to be? *Why?*

The letter arrived: No point in coming back, no point in upsetting the children again. No point. Happier separated. House gone. Furniture stored. No point coming back to Canada. So the bags were unpacked, the ticket money refunded. We stayed at my parents' house a little longer, then I started looking for a flat, answering ads. It was an amazing experience.

Firstly, the standard of flats in Dublin in 1965. You could call any space a flat, charge what you liked and impose any conditions on a tenant. They were damp, dirty, offering minimal facilities, and landladies — I didn't meet a landlord for some time — seemed to have no awareness that the space they rented was intended as a home. They wanted deposits and references, and then the question: where was my husband? When I said I was separated and here on my own, they didn't want to know. This was after I had been able to convince them that my children were too big to be destructive and that I wasn't likely to have a baby. One woman, standing beside a picture of the Sacred Heart in her hallway, said: "I'd rather not have a woman of your sort in the house."

Another woman said she'd rent me what was only

slightly better than a slum if I got a letter from my father's solicitor saying he would guarantee the rent. Yet another woman asked my religion, and when I said Jewish, she replied: "Well, you people pay your bills, anyway, but I'll have to ask my husband what he'd think." I took to travelling around looking at flats with a wad of notes in my bag. It worked. Eventually I got a place in Orwell Road. That I moved into it at all must have had quite a lot to do with masochism. It was a basement, dreary and damp as only a Dublin basement can be. We didn't stay long. The landlady tormented herself with the idea of what the children could, would or might do to her property — her main concern was the garden. Their disturbance of the gravel as they ran into the driveway from school caused her frenzy, and every time they ventured outside at the week-end she was there to warn them off the grass or down from the trees. She would have preferred it if I had not been around either, walking on her floors, sitting on her gruesome furniture. In fact she was a caricature of the wicked landlady. She wanted the money without having the bother of tenants at all and when I left the flat I suggested sarcastically that of course I would continue to send her rent.

Irish people do seem to have a problem with being fair to tenants. I found few who grasped the fact that their property was someone else's home after they had rented it, and constant territorial song and dances made life difficult. A race memory of colonialism? Perhaps.

In relation to that particular landlady, the very walls of her dismal basement seemed to reject our presence, and I was only in the place a week before I started looking for somewhere less punitive. I found a decent flat at last, three minutes from my parents' house. It was one side of the lower part of "Moyola", a fine old house in its own grounds on the lower Churchtown road. It was owned by the hotelier and developer P.V. Doyle, from whom I rented this home in peace and dignity for several years. Indeed on one occasion when maintenance had not arrived from Canada and I was short of money to pay the rent I rang him to explain. He told me not to worry and sent out a letter to that effect. "Attend to it when you can," said this famous Irish capitalist.

The flat was fairly well furnished and equipped and, although cold as hell under its fine Georgian ceilings, it had plenty of space inside and out. Nobody bothered the children, who were free to kick a ball or cycle a bike around the yard. The kitchen opened onto a little greenhouse in which grew a grape-vine, sour but profuse. There was an enormous living-room and two bedrooms. It felt like "home" at last.

Now I began to look for a job. I simply looked in the papers and answered the want ads. One job was that of a doctor's receptionist in Terenure. The doctor turned me down on the basis that I wouldn't stay. My husband would send for me, he said, how could a doctor be without a wife? Anyway, he said, I wasn't really the type for a doctor's surgery. He felt his patients would prefer an older, stouter woman, if I knew what he meant.

The next job was as a receptionist in a "health clinic". The man interviewing me seemed delighted when I walked into his office, then seemed to grow more and more uneasy. When he asked me if I'd ever done any massage and I said that I would be willing to learn he got very red in the face and said he would be in touch with me. On the bus going home I tried to figure out how I had messed up the interview.

Nobody wanted to give me a job, it seemed. I had reached rock-bottom when I applied for the post advertised in a firm set up to combat baldness. It was a sleazy, dandruffy sort of office. The man kept looking at my hair. Then he mentioned he had been hoping for someone a little younger. Then he asked me how I felt about bald men. Looking back, I realise that my total lack of revulsion to male baldness had a great deal to do with my not getting that job. Yes, of course I knew bald men, I said, but I hadn't really thought much about it ... Idiot. I ought to have curdled at the thought, said there should be a law against baldness. I believe the place is still in existence, employing very young women who view baldness as a personal insult.

I had been offered a job selling cosmetics in a chemist's shop when one of my old friends from my teens in the *Irish Times,* Sam Edgar, came up with the news that a new women's magazine was being started by Seán O'Sullivan and wouldn't I be great at it and why didn't I ring Seán and go and see him.

"Oh Sam ..." I said, feeling he didn't realise how incapable I was these days.

"Look, you know more about newspaper work than you do about cosmetics. A woman's magazine is only an expanded woman's page. Off with you. Selling cosmetics!"

It was true I knew nothing about cosmetics except that I used a lot of them. And if Sam Edgar, now dead, Lord rest him, thought I'd be any good to a magazine, well, hadn't he taught me most of anything I knew?

I got the job with *Irishwoman's Journal,* "the magazine for the thinking woman" and turned down the chemist's shop. I was taken on as assistant editor, a good title for a general dogsbody on a magazine run on a shoe-string. The year was 1965, the salary £7 a week and the hours, going and coming, were flexible. I didn't haggle about the pay. It meant I had got my foot back in the door of Irish journalism and I was over the moon.

Seán O'Sullivan is an American married to an Irish woman called Margaret, and he worked for Ireland's first woman's glossy magazine, *Creation.* He had this idea that there were a lot of thinking Irish women like his wife about whose interests in life were other than clothes or peeking into other women's dining-rooms. He was, of course, only fifteen years before his time. Women may have been thinking in Ireland in those days, but they had not yet found a voice. I, for one, was puzzled by the logo "thinking woman". What were they thinking *about?* In the meantime, the format of the magazine was the same as I had been used to in other magazines. There was fashion and beauty, a problem page, personalities, travel, a bit of coy comedy, cookery, knitting, fiction, and a controversial article, usually written by Seán O'Sullivan. The journal did well, although it would have done better with more capital, and I learned a great deal about magazine editing from Seán. He was the hardest-working man I had ever met in my life. No job was too small for him, no hour too late, no detail unworthy of attention. His respect for his readers was total. Any crazy wall-banger of a letter-writer would get the same personal painstaking reply as anyone else.

It was through talking to Seán, mostly over lunch in Bewley's of Grafton Street, that I began to develop confidence enough to give myself permission to live the way I wanted to live. I wasn't sure exactly what that entailed, except that there was no way I wanted to return to the housewife's cage again, to be isolated, cut off from the world and from myself. It took surprisingly little time, now that I had a satisfying interest, to look after the flat and the children's needs. There was always a pot of home-made chicken soup on the stove in case I was late getting home from a press reception or a natter with the girls in Searson's pub. I was beginning to enjoy my life, my independence. All I needed was a wife.

My luck still running, I found one, a mother of five children living right next door to me. She was a great "wife" to me, always helpful, cheerful, supportive and sympathetic and her older children baby-sat if need be. She freed me, for a while, from all the little worries that had filled up my head for years. Take the garbage out, buy more socks, decide what to have for dinner, boil the tea-towels, make school-lunches, scrub the lavatory. If she was there when I got home, she handed me a cup of tea.

She was only with me a couple of years, before she moved house, but in that time I learned, the easy way, that freedom was not the prerogative of men and that slavery for women was only as natural as their ability to accept it.

I wrote under three or four different names for the magazine. I was the fashion expert, the beauty expert and the problem page auntie. Apart from that I dealt with a lot of the contributors; I knew what women wanted from a magazine; after all, hadn't I absorbed the material for years? All women's magazine material (well, most of it) is simply a matter of re-hashing basic concepts. However, the fact that I had been reading international women's magazines rather than Irish ones caused me a lot of surprise, over the first year at any rate. For instance, contraception as a subject bored me stiff. Yet Seán O'Sullivan went on and on about it. To me, it seemed, he was obsessed with the subject and the Church's involvement in it. Always having had access to contraception in Ireland, it was difficult for me to believe, emotionally, that most women were in a bind about it. I couldn't quite understand the Catholic attitude. I couldn't appreciate why women didn't simply suit themselves and their own bodies, couldn't suppress the irritation I felt when bishops, doctors, priests and male journalists went on about contraception, felt vaguely impatient with Seán for writing about it. If it had to be written about, why not find a woman to do so? I still wasn't in the full of my health, of course, often feeling fearful and confused, but one thing I seemed to know in my bones was that a woman's body did not "belong" to any man or any body of men. That this could be permitted seemed to me a philosophy of slavery and even in my lack of feminist consciousness I felt great impatience with women who played such a silly game.

"I asked the priest if I could use the pill," a woman told me, "and he said no, so I'm off it again. I dread it, and then what when this baby arrives?"

Her letter stunned me on two counts, knocked me from side to side. I couldn't identify with her taking the priest's word for her sex life. How could such a morbid approach to sexuality be embraced in spiritual terms? And she'd said "I'm off it again", as if she hadn't anything to do with the whole business. The more I listened to people the more I realised that few took responsibility for their own sexuality. Sex was somehow so buried in shame and taboo that it was as if a spiritual condom protected the natural function of sexual intercourse from the reality of relationship. The effect of this gross condom was to separate people, especially women, so completely from their own sexuality that sex was always experienced as once removed. In fact, listening to married women talking about sex, when they did, I was convinced that a bowel movement was more real to them, more satisfactory, than sexual intercourse.

Alongside this I started to get very angry. Unwanted pregnancy, it seemed to me, was the ultimate slavery. To have one's body taken over for nine months, to be occupied unwillingly for that time, much less again and again, sickly, heavy, reluctant, trapped, having to face the pain and the aftermath and fear and then the same again within six weeks, seemed akin to crucifixion. All that suffering, indignity, oppression dismissed by being put into the context of the sanctity of Irish marriage brought for a long time only one word from me: "Yuck."

"Yuck," indeed. The quality of Irish life had begun to reveal itself to me. The hypocrisy, the double standards, the creepy-crawly self-righteous bullshit of the sixties was staggering. It wasn't that I was in a mood to judge. I was still smarting from my own misfortunes and willing to be tolerant and accepting. The fact was, though, that so many of the marriages I observed were clearly in a worse state than the one I had escaped. There was so much marital unhappiness, so many marriages awash with booze. For a while it seemed to me that unhappy marriage was more common here, but that is only, I suppose, that in Canada couples were not together by the time they would have got to that stage of mortal combat. I had few married couples among my friends, water finding its own level, but I had plenty of separated friends and friends who lived a separate life outside their marriages. Married men hunting for a bit on the side were so thick on the ground that often they impeded movement. They crowded the pubs where one ate or drank with pals, crowded the pubs to avoid going home. I wondered if their wives were as naive as I had been living in Ontario. And yet there wasn't much pub life there.

The classiest proposition I ever received there was from a fatherly tycoon who asked me to be his "lady" during his wife's unsafe period. He said it over a casual lunch, making the case calmly, firmly, proud of his honest approach. I shouldn't have thrown my drink in his eyes; it could have blinded him, I suppose.

I was relaxing in my slippers, hair in a towel, one night, when a State car complete with driver parked in front of my hall door. When I opened it, in staggered the totally intoxicated Minister whom I had interviewed the week before. He couldn't stand, but he had, he explained, looking for all the world like a skinned and over-heated toad, brought a "spot of supper" and "bubbly" for us. I felt sorry for the man, the father of a family who doubtless thought that he was working late as usual, for the greater good of his constituents.

"Look," I said to the driver, "take him off with himself."

The sober working man ignored me and proceeded to carry the basket of supper into my house.

"Right," I said, "I'll call the police and tell them a drunk has broken into my home."

"But he's a Minister of State," said the driver, "you can't treat him like that. Think of the scandal!"

"I don't care if he's a parish priest," I raved, "get that stuff back in the car and himself in along with it or you'll never get over the size of the scandal ..." With that we heard a thump and found the Minister flat-out inside my hall door. The driver dragged the unfortunate man out, stowed him in the back of the limo and glared at me before he took off. Two days later I received a massive bunch of flowers with no card, and was sure I knew where they came from.

Part, also, of this quality of Irish life were the number of women I met who had given babies away for adoption. I was astonished at the bland way they told their tales, sipping a gin and tonic, putting it all in the past, virgins once again on the hunt for husbands in a city which had so few eligible men. Their stories of how they had sneaked off to have their babies, their families never knowing, wrung my heart. Imagine that they hadn't been able to turn to a sister or an aunt, much less a mother, at such a time. Somehow, they foraged their way out of the miserable mess, the most important aspect of which was to keep it all secret.

The relief of not being found out kept them buoyed up for a couple of years. Often, it seemed to me, they convinced themselves that "it" had never happened. Certainly, the complete collusion of everyone around made it possible to bury the fact, in many cases, more deeply than could be healthy. To a girl — these eternal girls — they spoke about their first-borns with the same matter-of-fact briskness one uses having discovered that the hairdresser went scissor-happy while you dozed. "Water under the bridge. Probably all for the best."

Water under the bridge? Gone, but not forgotten. Never forgotten. Many's the picture of a new-born infant, now cracked and yellowed, kept in a secret place. Some of these convent girls, in their panic, had holed up in Dickensian baby homes, others hid out in London or elsewhere. Their parents never knew they had grandchildren, because they didn't want to know, and would have been terrified of knowing. Part of this quality of Irish life was the amazing ease with which it was possible to deceive parents, the ease with which these sheltered girls could drop out of their environment for months on end. Or the girl could be full-blown under their noses and they wouldn't see she was pregnant.

Such a case was a girl I'll call Mavis. When she was pregnant, she also got T.B. She spent the nine months in a sanatorium where she was visited regularly by her parents, but they never noticed she was pregnant. Never saw the child jump. As the months slipped by the nursing nuns arranged the bed-clothes in such a way as to disguise her belly. "I was huge," she told me. Then she had the child and signed it over to adoptive parents six weeks later. Her parents never knew. Times change, yet none too thoroughly, for nowadays that woman lives in suburbia, butter solid in her mouth. And the saddest thing of all, perhaps, is that if her own daughter were to become pregnant, the same denial system would quickly be brought into operation.

I never met an unmarried father. In fact, rarely did I hear the name of an unmarried father mentioned. Besides, a lot of them *were* married, to other women. What was a masculine sin? What could a fellow do that would cut him off from everything and everyone in shame and isolation? I didn't meet any middle-class men who went to jail, but heard of many a one who was a hard man. Any man's gross and irresponsible behaviour, in those days of the sixties, was reckoned to be excusable on the grounds that he was a "hard man", and had probably been too drunk to know what he was doing. The tolerance for drunken behaviour was amazing. To hold drunken behaviour over anyone the next day was considered unreasonable. "Ah sure, the poor bastard ..." For a while I got caught up in the vodka and soda cult myself. Even two drinks made me feel lousy, but gosh, the things I could get away with saying when I'd had a couple!

Not that it was ever permissible to behave like a man. A year after one girl gave her baby up for adoption, her family spent a goodly part of its capital defending the behaviour of her drunken brother before a court of law.

"You see," I said, "you should have trusted your parents, they'd have helped you, too."

"Not a chance," she shivered, "sex isn't the same as manslaughter, you don't understand. They'd have died of the shame." And the other women at lunch agreed. Rules, rules, tight little rules, and most of them — the inflexible ones at any rate — had to do with controlling women. And who was better at playing all the rules of oppression than these young women? They'd have jumped at anything to get a man to the altar, and some of them did. Some were waiting for years for Mammy's boys to make up their minds, and they wouldn't let go, couldn't let go. It might be a girl's last chance to get a husband. Indeed, her family had already begun to see spinsterhood as a reality, in the face of which words must be dropped in the right place by the influential uncle. From this powerful Irish activity, it was hoped, would come a permanent, pensionable job, next best thing to a husband.

"My mother is getting pretty desperate," Mavis told me, "she asked me how is it that a divorced Jewess like you can get an army captain and I've not a sign of anybody."

I was shocked by the mother's image of me, and sorry for Mavis that she felt she had to let me know about it. Anyway, I was having a thoroughly satisfying affair with the army captain. True, it was fraught with turbulence, Celtic twilight, and guilt (his), but that all contributed to the delicious neurosis of a passionate affair. I had found the most incredible sex object (him) and had I had the sense I'd have worried less and enjoyed it even more.

Meanwhile, I assured Mavis: "You will, I promise you, have a husband and children and live in a nice house in suburbia. And may the Lord have mercy on you." She looked relieved and grateful. I realised how sure I was of her future. It was just so obvious that if you want something so desperately that you'll make any deal with yourself to get it, are prepared to do anything to reach your goal and have society behind you to boot, well, then ...

And my friend was putting her all into her husband hunt. So were her peers. God, the bargains some of them landed, the beauties they manipulated away from the bar; the effort employed to prise the boys apart for as long as it took for a wedding and a honeymoon and that disappointed look traced on the face of the smiling housewife.

It made me cringe to see these fine young women try so hard for so little. I feel sad, nowadays, when we meet and they avoid my eyes. And yet, unmarried, what had they to look forward to? Perhaps it was just my luck to meet the desperate ones. Perhaps there were easy, happy relationships being formed all over the country. In any case, it's not as bad as that anymore, is it? Or is it?

The 'sixties were a good time for the boys. Lemass's Ireland was flourishing, business booming, high hopes. There was money around and employment and optimism. And if one had been a mite more sensitive, it would have been possible to recognise the anger that was mounting under the surface as the decade went on. It was female anger, subtle, veiled, but there. It was an anger the cause of which I only partly recognised or understood. It was a hang-over, an almighty international hang-over. It was an anger which clearly said: "OK, the awful 'fifties are gone, things are going right for a change. Going right for the boys. But what about us?" And the worst of the hang-over was trying to shake off the 'fifties, the weight of having been teen-agers in a decade which hadn't yet invented the teen-ager. Cocooned in marriage, I had skipped the 'fifties for all practical purposes, had been unaware of their oppression. They had been happy years for me, in love, with small babies. I was not aware of my status being that of a favoured slave.

I had looked with sympathy upon the oppression of the Red Indian, the American black, the Northern Ireland Catholic. Now here in Ireland I began to feel terribly, terribly angry.

"Ah well, it's because your marriage broke up," someone would say sympathetically.

6
ABORTION

I can feel the smooth sheets on my legs, the softness under my head and relief starts to seep through the headiness of the anaesthetic. My arm is cold. I feel it being lifted and covered. Sighing and snuggling down I'm satisfied that I don't have to get up. The freckled face of the nurse bends over me. I smile at her:

"Could I see my baby, please?" I ask.

A funny look comes over her face.

"Is it a girl or a boy? Let me see?"

Yes, she looks funny. Did she draw away from me? Oh God, something's wrong with my baby! I try to struggle up and gently she puts me back on the pillow.

"Please don't upset yourself," the accent is Irish, "it'll be alright. I'll be back in a tic." But I've recognised that look. Pity.

"What's wrong?" I call after her back. "You can tell me, just tell me?" I lie back on the pillow exhausted. I must be near the labour ward, a cubicled little space. I'm on one of those trolley things. They haven't taken me to my room yet. The nurse is back with someone else on the other side of the bed. The panic makes my throat feel squeezed. I gasp for breath. His two heads say:

"June, come now. What appears to be the trouble?"

Trouble? Hasn't she told him? I look at her. She has told him. Stupid man. I say with peevish irritation, the best I can muster by way of an order:

"Get my baby, will you? I want to see ..."

That smell, that smell that warns of power approaching. Now the nurse's gentle hand is holding my arm and rubbing the smelly icyness over the cracks inside my elbow.

"Just a prick," whispers the nurse from Limerick to coincide with the sting. "Yes," I think, "aren't they all?" And I go sailing downwards, wanting to stay, down down, but here I am again, softly in a cosy bed, scent of roses, that familiar nurse sitting by my bed. She looks concerned. Had I given them trouble?

"Hello," she says, "are you feeling better now?" I remember I've been having an abortion in a London clinic. I'm not pregnant any more. And I remember the rest.

"Yes," I said, smiling a bit tearfully, "I'm feeling relieved. Sorry to have given you such a hard time." She squeezed my hand.

That is how it was for me.

On the 'plane back to Dublin, my life seemed given back to me. A-a-hh, the relief, the wonderous relief. I was not pregnant, not pregnant, not pregnant. Now I understand why so many an Irish lass returned from England to disport herself as a virgin once again. The elation of a second chance. A clean slate. Yes, I'd broken laws, but I was going home free. The relief. I thought my prayers were being answered. It did occur to me, after I calmed down, that I might have something to explain to that Person. I'd think about that later.

Journalist Mary Holland, some time ago, called upon women like me to send their names to a list she, herself, headed for publication in Dublin's *Hibernia*, the excellent weekly review which is no more. A list of women who'd had abortions. Her request was greeted with silence. In a social climate such as ours what is the point of having an abortion if you are going to tell people about it? I don't much care what people think. Those who grasp at any reason to blame, to condemn, will find a way of doing so anyway. Others couldn't care less. And then there are those others who like to know the truth to widen their awareness of a subject.

After I joined the women's movement, I realised that I must some day share my abortion experience in an effort to help others to think the problem through. But I needed time in which to think it out myself, first. For all the radical image of that first group, they never got round to discussing abortion, not even in consciousness raising. I didn't say anything because I had so many feelings to unravel. I didn't write to Mary Holland because I didn't want to risk my truth by signing away the fact.

"June Levine is pro-abortion, she had one herself," may still be said. At least I've tried to shed a bit of light. I am anti-abortion, but I had to have one myself. I'm telling it the way it was for me in the hope of helping someone else figure how it might be for her. Before, rather than later. That's important.

In the 'sixties I reacted against being pregnant with every cell of my body, every hair of my head. I did not want to have a baby. I could not face carrying it through nine months of vomiting and poor health. I did not want to go through child birth. Also, at that stage I could not have supported my family on what I earned and I felt quite sure that my alimony would be stopped when it was learned I was pregnant. I did not want to start rearing another infant.

Since the beginning of time women have tried to abort themselves. Long before men told them about sin. Before men got into the abortion business. Women managed in weird ways long before and far away from abortionists or even gin and hot baths. Primitive women have used everything from weeds and clay stuffed up their vaginas to poisons and spells. I knew a woman who upon finding herself pregnant insisted on vigorous sex with her husband all through a holiday, day and night, hour after hour. It worked, it seems. He told her: "I'll never go through that again."

The abortion trail from Ireland to England is not a fresh one. It did not result from the British abortion laws being changed in the late 'sixties. Irish women have always gone to England for abortions. Most had back street abortions.

Who would risk a back street abortion unless the alternative was even more terrifying and impossible? And yet many an Irish woman has gone to English back-street abortionists not simply because abortion wasn't available to them otherwise, but also because they were paying out of a woman's insufficient pay packet. I paid through the reluctant father's nose. He was friendly about it, insisted on paying the full whack, about £600 at the time. If he hadn't, I couldn't. I'd have gone for something more risky.

Let's go back to the beginning. I had no unconscious motive for getting pregnant. I say that to clear the air. In Ireland, it seems, women often think of pregnancy as punishment for sexual activity. Such a woman may very well bring about her own "punishment" while overtly practicing birth control. Accident. Makes her sub-conscious feel better. And of course there are women who want to be pregnant, but use contraception because they feel they should.

I don't happen to regard sex between consenting adults as an occasion for punishment. Sex is not one of my guilt triggers. I had no unconscious urge to be "found out". Nor did I wish for another child. So, the secondary cause of my pregnancy was ignorance. Reasonable ignorance.

I was on the Pill. It had always worked for me. I would have thought my ovaries were pretty shell-shocked. I went to the doctor and told him I thought I was pregnant.

He said: "You can't be unless you forgot to take your pill. Did you forget?"

"No, but I'm pregnant. I know it."

"Even if you weren't on the pill, you couldn't possibly know it yet."

Oh, couldn't I? What was the use of arguing!

Now, I know that you can get pregnant while you are on the pill. Depends what else you are on. How many doctors, especially those working outside of family planning clinics, warn their patients of the Pill's possibility of interacting with other drugs? Pregnancy in pill users is often put down to stupidity or carelessness. Many general practitioners in Ireland dispense contraceptive advice, mainly the pill, without having any special training. Some drugs prescribed for ailments do interact with the pill. Many Irish women, myself included, came by this information only when it was published in the first edition of the *Irish Women's Diary*, produced in 1980 by *Irish Feminist Information*, set up by Róisín Conroy. They printed a chart from *Spare Rib*. Drugs which can interact with the pill are certain antibiotics and some of the drugs which act on the nervous system. At the time I became pregnant I was taking prescribed antibiotics and "nerve pills".

"I think you ought to ask yourself," said my doctor, "why you forgot to take your pill?" I searched for the missing pill or pills. If I hadn't swallowed them as usual, where in hell were they? Meanwhile, I was pregnant. It couldn't happen, but it had.

As soon as I mentioned pregnancy to a friend or two I was snowed under with information about where to get an abortion. The most unlikely people had information. I didn't need an abortion referral agency. In fact, I was so flooded with information, I couldn't decide ...

A positive effect of the abortion debate in Ireland has been forcing people to admit that abortion happens; hopefully the debate also helps women think things out a bit less simplistically. However, I recall, it did not occur to any of the women to whom I spoke in those pre-women's liberation days that I might not have an abortion. They *knew* it was what I would have to do. Who were they, these women? Most of them would have been under thirty, working girls because back then there were very few married women working. One or two would have been journalists, most would be secretaries or in jobs of a similar nature. Through them I heard of other women, friends of theirs, cousins. And in Dublin's swanky lounges of the "swinging sixties" I heard of another kind of Irish woman who availed of abortion in England. She was the glamorous wife of the upwardly mobile man of the 'sixties. These women were not legion, but they did exist. A young woman took leave of her husband for a shopping spree in London and returned "honeymoon fresh". That was the phrase.

Suddenly, in my predicament, everyone seemed to know about abortion. The other surprising thing was that now the fact of having had a child adopted was being related to me in the same context. Every day or so there were these little explosions of confidences: "I had to give a baby up for adoption," or "I had an abortion." I was one of the girls.

"Look," said the co-parent, "it's important to get the right man for the job. Leave it to me."

We were sitting in the Shelbourne Bar. Just at that moment, he spotted someone on the other side of the bar:

"Just a sec," and off he went.

When he came back he had got "perfect information" from another Irish Catholic father. I strained my neck to have a better look at the source.

"It's OK," I was told, "he's a reliable type. Has seven kids."

The rich are different, I recalled from Scott Fitzgerald, not just because they have money. My biological state seemed to reflect the lowliness of my status.

"I suppose," I asked wanting to cause consternation, "I could change my mind and go through with it?"

"Ah now, Amigo," that was the trendy name for people you were screwing around with that year, "I have to think of my family."

"This is your family," I said with the bland face I reserve for jugular attacks. I never even bothered to observe my target. The thrust had boomeranged, leaving me with an awful awareness. The thought obsessed me, tormented me, but my desperation drove me on. Another child now would wipe me out. I could imagine every miserable awful day of what lay ahead and the circumstances. Abortion was a raft. I was terrified of that raft, but ...

The "right person" turned out to be three people. All of them in or around Harley Street. Two of the doctors were psychiatrists. The law in Britain then allowed a woman an abortion if two psychiatrists would say it would dangerously damage her mental health if she went on through childbirth. I felt that this was accurate in my case. Even so, it was a formality, I was assured, but first I had to see the obstetrician. I went along to his little terraced house off Harley Street, stopping en route from Heathrow Airport, to check my suitcase into the hotel. It was all very, very unreal. As if I were playing a part in a film. I felt this vague interest in what was going to happen next. It seemed to me that the whole city of London was expecting me, waiting for me.

I was not at all surprised by the mundane shabbiness of the doctor's rooms. To me, it would have seemed more real if they had smelled of cabbage and the elderly receptionist had worn a blood spattered coat. As it was, she was a "no frosting on *this* cake" type, plump, tweedy, dismissive. She sat in a little cubicle at the bottom of the hall, under the stairs. I could see her cup of tea on the little table, barely leaving room for her chair. There was an electric bar fire beneath it and I looked down at her legs to see if she had ABC marks on them, but she wore thick stockings.

"Why are you here?" she asked me, barely short of rudeness. "Have you an appointment with the doctor?"

"I'm from Dublin," I said quietly not wanting to start anything, "the doctor is expecting me."

"Ah yes," she said loudly, "the maternity case from Dublin. The doctor is very busy, but he'll get to you this afternoon."

I followed her into a waiting room. Memory does strange things. The room was packed with women, young women. What I remember most clearly is the brownness. Brownness descended about my brain, that afternoon. Even the air seemed brown in that brown room with brown furniture and brown clothes. No blonde hair, no fair skin, no light eyes. I seem to remember I was wearing brown. Yet it could not be so. I never wore brown. Black is my dark colour.

I became part of the bogginess, sitting on the edge of an arm chair in which another brown woman sat in her brown space. Nobody looked at anyone else. Nobody looked pregnant. No taut bulges. I remember I could not give that thought time in my head to come up with a logical answer.

Eventually, the room emptied to a comfortable crowd, weeded systematically by the brown receptionist.

"There's been a mistake," she said to me, "you should have gone in when you arrived." I followed her into another waiting-room packed with women. Another brown-filled room.

I walked through the brownness, feeling the prickle of eyes on my back and then I was in a small bright surgery. At the desk opposite the door, sat a small, plump balding blonde man, tired, ordinary. He was on the 'phone.

No, he couldn't make it before seven thirty. Yes, oh that sounded good. No, he thought maybe blue. Yes, quite right. No, something light would do. See you later. Take care.

I was surprised when he spoke because he had absolutely no medical manner at all. Not a trace. Practical man. A one to one approach, like a grocer or an electrician. Relieved, I took my tiny tissue-wrapped bottle out of my bag and handed it to him.

"What is this?" he asked, before he realised.

"It's for you," I said, "I thought you'd like it."

"Thank you," he said politely, not looking me in the eye and placing the bottle on the desk, "let's see what we are talking about here." He beckoned to the chair. I went behind the small screen and took off my coat and knickers. The examination took about five seconds.

"Yes," he said peeling off his gloves, "definitely. Were you using anything?"

"The pill."

He looked irritated. "I see. Look, if I fix you up you'll have to take the pill in future. I won't do it twice."

I nodded.

He came to the point. "I want you to come back in two weeks time with two envelopes. One hundred and twenty pounds in each for the psychiatrists and the clinic fee. Cash. Bank notes only. Is that a problem?"

I shook my head. My throat had seized up again.

"When you come back, you'll see the psychiatrists and I'll fix things. Don't forget the envelopes. They insist on being paid first."

"Of course," I said, "Of course." I was a-quiver with gratitude. Then a thought struck me:

"Suppose they won't agree to sign?" I asked. His face cleared as if in recognition of something. Probably the fact that he had a right wet standing opposite him.

"They will," he said and then kindly: "They will. Look at yourself. Of course they'll sign. Try to relax. It'll be fine."

I let out a long sigh to show him I was relaxed and brownly made my way back through the brownness. From there I went back to the hotel room and lay on the bed in the burning central heat, amazed at how far I'd got, too nauseated to take my clothes off and aware that my kidney trouble was beginning as in other pregnancies.

Two weeks later I was back in London, all orders carried out. I rang the obstetrician.

"You have the envelopes?"

"Yes."

"The money for the clinic?"

"Yes, of course."

"Now, go to ..." and he gave me an address. "They are both in the same building, but you have an appointment to see Dr. M. first. He'll send you on ..."

The first psychiatrist was a "man of the world", cocktail-party mannered man.

I'd been married to a doctor? Well, well, they would have to do the best they could for me, wouldn't they? Did I work? Ah, a journalist. I wouldn't write about them, would I? I wasn't playing a little joke was I? Heh, heh, heh, a journalist would do anything for a scoop these days. Wasn't that what it was called, a scoop?

"What?" I asked, horrified. Why must he use words like "scoop"? Better not point that out. Never know how he might turn. He was smoothing things out now. Taking my envelope, holding my coat, bowing, directing me to the other doctor on another floor. I was feeling confused, humiliated, with that awful anger rising through the rest. Then he remembered they had to do the best for me, so he *escorted* me to the second psychiatrist. He introduced us, backed away a little as if in the presence of royalty and took his leave.

Honestly, the second man looked like Sigmund Freud. He was a foreigner too. Jewish. We clashed on sight. I knew he despised me. I merely hated him.

"You are a churnalist?" he asked.

"Yes," I agreed, "but I am not writing about this."

"Vy not? *I* should know you vill not?"

"How can I?" I was astonished by this turn of events. "Do you think I would get pregnant just so I could write a story about ..."

"So! *I* should know vy you get pregnant?" He went on in the same vein. He ranted about why women got pregnant and expected him to undo their stupidity. I was getting more and more frightened. He wasn't going to sign. What would I do if he said No?

"How do I know you vill not tell your husbunt? Vhere he is anyvay? I don't *care* vhere he is ..."

I had started to cry, but I noticed he had the white envelope in his hand, was tapping it on the desk. You bastard, I thought, you want that money. You'll probably hold on to it anyway.

"Vhat vould your husbunt sink off zis?" he was asking me. I was suddenly in a wild rage, mimicking his accent, spitting each word out on a breath of its very own: "If you don't *vont* to sign, give me back the money, because if you vill *not* I will tell *every-bloody-body* ..."

He was furious. He bundled me out, told me that Dr. S. the obstetrician would hear from him. I was in the taxi on my way to the clinic when I realised he had the envelope. Ah, so he was going to do it? Maybe not. God, what a shit.

I was sitting in the comfortable suburban looking bedroom in the clinic with the Irish nurse when the obstetrician arrived. He looked hassled:

"Dr. F. doesn't feel happy about you ..."

I didn't let him finish. "You think I'm going to elope

with *him?*" His expression softened: "I've told him he is being over-cautious. What did you say to him? He said you insulted him?"

Suddenly, unexpectedly, my teeth started to chatter. I clinched my jaws together, but I shook uncontrollably and the nurse ran across the room and held me in her arms as if to hold my bones together. "I just hate doctors. I h-h-hate doc—tors," I said pressing into her arms. "I h-hate him. He's a, he's, he's — a-lousy-old-goat." He just stood there, looking at me and the Irish nurse went on cradling, murmuring, stroking until I calmed. Then suddenly, I had to break away from her to vomit.

The doctor stood at the bathroom door.

"Are you alright?" he asked.

"Lovely," I said flatly.

"We don't usually have this sort of thing happen," he said.

"Neither do I," I said wearily, "all my other abortions have been delightful."

He sort of smiled: "Look, *I* think you are on the level. Don't worry, Dr. F. will sign. You see he thinks you might be a bit unstable."

It was years later it dawned on me that I'd paid those men to say I was "too unstable".

I was being wheeled into the theatre next morning, on my way at last, when I became aware of the obstetrician walking alongside me.

"I'm RH negative," I said dopily, "I was told not to have another child ..."

He squeezed my hand: "Stop worrying. Dr. F. signed. There's only me now."

* * *

Memories come when I think of abortion. Childhood memories of an atmosphere charged with tension, fear, mystery. And femaleness. Central to the atmosphere there was the awareness of a special "something" that threatened women. Something not seen, not understood by men and children. It was something I knew all women had in common. It was an important something that you spoke about in whispers. Because of that "something" I remember now, at different stages in my childhood I was aware that my mother or an aunt or some other woman was hugely worried.

I remember wanting to know what the "something" was and yet not wanting to know. I can feel the threat of it now and my fascination with that atmosphere. The "something" threatened worse than not having money, bigger than a fight with a husband. It was even bigger, certainly closer, than the fear that Hitler might come to Ireland. And yet, it never seemed to happen, this terrible something. A neighbour said she'd jump in the Liffey if it did. She didn't jump in the Liffey. I remember well she didn't because she had a new baby ages after she said that, so I remember she didn't. I often thought of the Liffey when I saw her baby. Somehow, as a child, the baby reminded me of the Liffey. I loved and feared the Liffey when I stood at the concrete wall near Capel Street bridge, looking into the dark wetness with my Grandy John. The Liffey was a long way from where we lived; you'd have to go all that way to jump in and then you'd be dead for sure. And yet it was better than that awful "something" happening.

I can remember at about ten years old feeling quite nauseated by that sense of something. I am standing beside two women in aprons. I have been told to go and mind the younger children, but I am stuck to the spot, fascinated. I make as if I'm going to go, but stay and put on a disinterested look. One neighbour is saying: "... nearly skinned the backside off myself, but I stuck it and when I got out I was dizzy from the heat. Wouldn't you think that'd work unless I'm gone?" The other woman says it's desperate. "Himself will be raging," says the first woman.

Ah, that "something" again. I know that voice. That feel. So her husband doesn't know about it either. "Himselves" are greatly to be feared. They seem to be more fearful than Daddies. Still, the woman doesn't seem really afraid of himself. She says: "Pity about him. The thought of facing it again. I'll be up in the Gorman, that's where I'll be." Her face is all screwed up and she looks awful.

The Gorman, I knew, was where mothers were driven by wild boys and other unbearable things: the big mental hospital, Grangegorman, somewhere in Dublin. You knew you'd pushed your mother to the limit when she said she'd end up in the Gorman. I asked my mother that night why our neighbour said she'd be going to the Gorman. Mammy said it was only talk. Still, I knew "something" was in the air. Poor Mrs. Quinn was worried. Even my mother admitted that. The woman's sons were driving her mad, they were that bold. I thought I might tell the boys that their mother was only waiting for something to happen and she'd be off to the Gorman. It was on the tip of my tongue to tell them when they were horse playing and knocked me on the ground, but I stopped in time. I knew that something that had Mrs. Quinn worried sick was not for male ears. Somehow, I knew. Anyway, they wouldn't understand. It gave me great satisfaction to think that my brothers would never be women. They'd never know. I'd know some day because I'd be a woman. I nearly knew now. Of course, you just grow into an awareness of the "something", ease into the reality of that female atmosphere, within the whispers, misery of sisterhood, the sisterhood beyond misery.

Later, I was amazed at how D.H. Lawrence empathised with Mrs. Morel trapped by another pregnancy in her struggle with poverty and ugliness and meanness. A mere man, he managed to just about approach that essence of fear and desperation which clung about Mrs. Quinn that day in the feared predicament. And so in my time I felt at one with Mrs. Quinn and Mrs. Morel and all women and yet alone, isolated. The "something" had stalked me down, calling forth the Gorman, the River Liffey. Worse. "Mrs. Quinn" (although that's not her real name) may remember me hanging around, as a child, to hear what she was saying. I wonder how she will feel if she reads about my trip to England. Probably, it depends on whether she allows herself trips to the past, back to the space we shared as women of different generations.

I admit to being shocked when Ann Connolly, who set up Dublin's Well Woman Clinic, stood before the nation voicing that women must have the right to choose abortion. It was as if, I too, would rather pretend that Irish women were not having abortions in their thousands every year. Women have always risked their lives to become unpregnant. All around me, in Dublin, are women who have had abortions or given babies up for adoption. It is amazing that there are so many of my age, older. All before the word was spoken aloud. Abortion. The right to choose? Who would have thought of such a thing? We had the right to be obedient wives or a-sexual creatures and beyond that we saw ourselves as failures, accepting the blame, the burden and the oppressive pain of shame. When as young wives or lovers we discussed something of a sexual nature we did so in half-truths, always in an atmosphere of bleak denial. Our psyches shuffled around like slaves doing what was expected, not wanting to be noticed by the master, or being noticed, desperately wanting reward. It never dawned on us that there might some day be an abolition of slavery, whether sexual, economic or otherwise. And that this abolition could come about by our own hands? It was hard to imagine that, since the Ku Klux Klan we most dreaded were the women who had absorbed the bosses' image of them. These sisters were our gallows-builders and it is those women, among them some of our very own mothers, whom we most feared. They had the power to invalidate us by their acceptance as "natural" and proper of the way things were. Who, above all, is more frightening, hurtful, than the one of us who identifies with the oppressor, bears witness to our transgressions by measuring them against her own "normality"?

Maureen has been my friend for years and years. I didn't tell her I'd had an abortion until one day she told me that she'd had one at age 22. Before that, she'd given a baby up for adoption. (Obviously, Maureen isn't her real name).

"Once is bad enough," it's been said. "Twice you need your head examined." Women like Maureen would probably spare themselves a second experience if they got a bit of feminist counselling first time round. The second time is now recognised by psychiatrists and therapists as a grief thing, the mother's unconscious attempt to replace the child lost through adoption or abortion.

Maureen, a Mayo girl, had wanted to be a lawyer, but her father felt university fees for a girl a waste of money. Instead, she went off to London at the age of nineteen to study drama by day, sometimes, and do all kinds of jobs to earn a crust by night. Like so many 'fifties Irish emigrants for England, Canada and America, she was ill-equipped for life by our insular education and sexual ignorance.

Predictably, Maureen became pregnant. She lived in a home for unmarried mothers before the birth, and was convinced she must have the child adopted by the horror stories that were told to her about girls who had tried to keep their babies. She was also introduced, by the matron of the home, to a few single mothers. She was shocked by the hardship of their lives and their prospects for child rearing. She parted with her son. Knowing her now, I cannot imagine a worse decision, given her personality. A strong woman with major survival techniques, the child would have been her pride and joy. All she needed was a bit of practical help, guidance, a leg up. She was not encouraged to think about keeping her infant. Nor had she ever been encouraged to believe in herself.

She recalls being visited by her father, the baby's grandfather, when she was pregnant: "I didn't know where to put myself. When he looked at me in that condition I felt so ashamed. I wanted to disappear. He didn't suggest that we should keep the baby. I couldn't imagine how we would do that."

She was soon pregnant again. She wasn't using contraception. This attitude to contraception seems peculiarly Irish Catholic, the "take a chance, but don't premeditate" thinking that may have something to do with the experience of Confession. Sin, it seems, can happen to a bishop but premeditated sin is mortal. People brought up in convent schools seem to have great difficulty with that one, like little children hiding their eyes to make themselves invisible.

In any case Maureen could not face the home a second time. A friend told her of an abortionist. Together, one night, they went to a shabby part of East End London and the doctor stuffed Maureen's vagina with soaked packing which he said would bring "it" on. It did not work and when she went back, he gave her an anaesthetic there and then and scraped her uterus.

Three days later, Maureen in her bed-sitter, developed a terrible chill and high temperature. Her friend called a doctor. He said no, he wouldn't come, call the hospital. Maureen remembers herself on fire, pushing the blanket off and the East End accent of the ambulance man saying: "Look, you better realise you are dying, young lady, keep that blanket on." He left her in the back of the ambulance and sat with the driver.

In the hospital, Maureen was treated punitively and dismissively. An abortion case. Serve her right. But finally, they got her well. They badgered her for the name of the abortionist. She wouldn't tell. Finally, before she left hospital, they told her she was still pregnant.

At home again, Maureen told her girl-friend that she was still pregnant. The other young woman knew that she was not.

Now the doctor who had refused to come helped. He told them that the hospital was expecting that Maureen would lead the police to him if she thought she was still pregnant. She would be followed for weeks.

Eventually Maureen got married, but suffered seven years of sterility for which there was absolutely no reason that the best Dublin obstetricians could find. She went from one doctor to another, but never told anyone of them of her London experience.

"The doctors kept telling me that they could find nothing wrong," she says, "but I knew it was the abortion. Or at least I thought I knew, but at the same time I couldn't tell them. Maybe, if I could have said it out loud I could have got pregnant."

It is medically accepted that sterility is sometimes the

result of hysteria caused by trauma.

The last decade has seen radical change in the position of the unmarried mother in Ireland, largely thanks to organisations like Cherish and Ally. The introduction of an unmarried mother's allowance has been accompanied by far greater social acceptance of the mother and her baby. Legislation has been introduced to make dismissal on the grounds of pregnancy "unfair", and those religious schools or hospitals which might still seek to sack an unmarried mother can be taken to a tribunal.

The reality of the situation is that housing, finance and child-minding are still major considerations for a single mother. Socially, the unmarried woman is more accepted, but commonly she may not bring her child to visit grandparents for fear of what the neighbours may think.

Women will always have unplanned pregnancies. And women have feelings about being pregnant besides those related to economic and social pressures. Some women have medical reasons, having come in contact with German measles, radiation treatment, and so on. Other women feel that they simply cannot face pregnancy and childbirth, whatever about what follows. In Ireland, the happy pregnancy is like the happy marriage. We conspire to believe that it is the "norm". Therefore we have little understanding of the compulsive action of many women to escape from pregnancy. Abortion is illegal and unavailable in Ireland. That hasn't stopped women going to England. If the proposed anti-Abortion Amendment to the Irish Constitution, to protect the life of the unborn, is passed through referendum, it will not stop Irish women going to England for abortions. It will be a slogan to further facilitate our tendency to act like the child who covers her eyes in an attempt to make herself invisible.

Who can be "for" abortion? I've worked it over, worked it through in an attempt to work it out of my system. For many women abortion is the instinctive escape from the ultimate female experience of being cornered, trapped, defeated. That's how it was with me. I was in that state where to go ahead with having another child would have meant "the Gorman". All that was before the women's movement came to Ireland, long before I met any of those liberated women, long before I met Mary Kenny.

7
WOMEN'S PAGE

Memories of the first day I met Mary Kenny make me smile. She does not recall that first encounter of ours at all, except that she thought I was "a nice lady". Typical of Mary — quaint expression, kind manners. The sun was shining and she sat astride a bicycle, skirting the kerb outside the Intercontinental Hotel, while I walked slowly along making last-minute arrangements for her to send copy to the *Irishwoman's Journal*. After lunch with me, she was on her way to "Gainsborough", a rambling old Georgian house, five minutes away, where her mother, Ita, widow of a diplomat, would pat her hair and refresh her lipstick before answering the hall-door.

Mary was wearing shorts and high heels and the famous legs always come into my mind when I see "Sindy" dolls in the toy shops at Christmas.

"My mother hates shorts, but doesn't everybody's mother?" and she flashed the wide grin to show there was no slight intended to her mother. "It's worse for her when I come home with a ladder in my stocking and she knows I've been *seen* like that, maybe in Grafton Street, for heaven's sake. That drives her crazy. She'd like me to dress like a lady, y'know, white gloves and hat."

She confessed to dressing like a lady in Paris with her mother. "It's a small thing and we have such a lovely time," she explained, making it sound as if white gloves and hats were *the* things which came between the generations; only for lack of compromise over trivia, we'd all be having a ball in Paris with our mothers.

Mary was twenty-three years old then. She fascinated me, being the walking fantasy of my youthful dreams, the potential image of myself I had abandoned. She cut a dashing figure. Free, white and over twenty-one, as they say in Dublin. I'd never felt free, never been aware of "whiteness" because of being half-Jewish, and as for being of age, I had only begun to think in my thirties of what that implied. Some pressure seemed to want to prevent me coming of age, ever. It was like an iron curtain blocking me from adulthood.

Mary was, at least, living out the illusion of being free and adult. Independence shone from her. She bounced around Europe working for the *Evening Standard*, drank in Fleet Street pubs with people who wrote the Sunday columns. Why did she want to work for the *Irishwoman's Journal?*

"Money," she replied, flashing the smile again. No-one talked as bluntly about money in those days. Then her face settled and she trusted me with: "Well actually, I'm easing my foot in the door here. Free-lancing won't do any harm if I want to come home." She was ambitious and admitted to ambition. She was totally different, in this respect, from the typical Irish girl, who would have been as embarrassed to have her ambition show as to have her knickers flutter grubbily around her ankles in Grafton Street.

I well remember how the confident thrust of her personality made me feel world-worn, depressed about starting all over again so late. Her energy was at once daunting and a turn-on. Her obvious rebelliousness ran like a river through the landscape of her personality, seemingly contained, constructive. Here was someone who was going to do more for herself than fret about the system and struggle halfheartedly with "the inevitable". As she rode off on her bike, I knew at last that the big mistake to make in life is to go around asking for permission. Whether permission was sought from other people, society or one's voices didn't matter. To ask for permission was to be shot down.

Mary simply forged ahead.

Mary was the sort of girl nuns warned their girls about. She was the kind of girl nuns dreaded. Mary was FORWARD. It was an impossible thing for an Irish convent girl to be, but she sussed pretty early that her only hope of escaping the life plan the nuns had in store for her was to be as forward as hell. Actually, the nuns did turn out a ladylike young woman in Mary, amusingly so, but the lovely manners were probably more a symptom of warm-heartedness and home environment than instruction. In Mary, the nuns attempted to rear a good Irish Catholic wife for some decent man. Good Catholic wife she may be, but she married an English Protestant, Richard West, the journalist and writer.

The nuns had tried to equip her for the appropriate job and her appropriate station in life. Forwardness, they made it plain, would ruin everything. Forward girls were brash and ugly and socially unacceptable. Nobody wanted a forward girl. Not boys, certainly, who would be concerned with finding a suitably demure mother for their future families. The nuns didn't want a forward girl around the place, asking impossible questions, being unseemly, stirring things up. Parents dreaded the forwardness of a daughter. Such a girl was unfeminine, a poor bet on the marriage market.

Mary realised that if you wanted to go forward there was no point in being backward. She felt put down by the elitist education given her, irked by the incessant emphasis on chastity and meekness and being demure. The nuns were snobs too. "I rebelled against a very Irish background of being female in the 'fifties. It was incredibly repressive. I knew there was a battle going on to keep me down. I'd been told by the nuns that I could be a shorthand typist and get into Guinness's if I was lucky, or I could be a teacher or a nun. Out of eighteen girls in my sister's class of 1956, sixteen became secretaries. It occurred to me to wonder why nobody ever said that you could become an architect or an accountant or a doctor, you know, and I felt held down. Not that the 'fifties were great for anybody. Lots of people were emigrating. There weren't enough jobs for the men, not to mind the women, to use an Irish expression ..."

So when she was eighteen she went to France as an *au pair* girl and wrote pieces for the *Evening Press* and the *Irish Times*. She collected a lot of cuttings and she remembered what the nuns had told her about not looking for notice. "I looked for as much notice as possible. If you're not pretty and you're not very well educated, you haven't been to Eton, you don't have any particular assets when you start in the world, you've got to do something. Some gimmick, and so I was a very forward, cheeky Irish girl."

She got a job as a secretary on the *Guardian* in London, and then she went to the *Evening Standard* and told the editor: "You've got to hire me because if you don't you really will miss something big." And he said: "Well, I can't possibly resist you if you feel like that. Miss Kenny, you are hired."

Now, in the Intercontinental Hotel, Dublin, we talked about ideas for articles. She was full of ideas but the first piece, we decided, would be about the female biological pressure to reproduce. In a word, Mary's urge to have a baby. We discussed biological urges as if we had invented them; I had never spoken about sex or urges or any such mysteries with another woman. Mary observed the primitive in herself objectively and I was relieved to be able to communicate, at last, my female "secret". At a certain time of the menstrual cycle, we agreed, there was always this fierce urge to become pregnant. Obviously, it was not during the safe period recommended by the rhythm method of birth control. She was aware of the danger, she told me, of how easy it would be to become an unmarried mother.

All this seems obvious stuff now, Mother Nature as the Boss Lady. All the freely available contraception in the world wouldn't work of its own volition. The Boss Lady will get her way unless she is foxed in your head first, not half-heartedly blocked down there where She thrives. And I thought these feelings peculiar to myself?

I had become bored by the subject of contraception. Now I saw that the reason was that the discussion never seemed to have anything to do with sexuality, with sex, with reality, the Boss Lady. Nor did I encourage Mary to write about contraception. I knew well only priests and married men could get away with such topics. And yet here was the beginning for me of a new type of journalism for women. This would be the reportage of subjective reality rather than the external happenings of the day. Rumours of the Women's Movement in America had started to filter through, but we did not speak of it, nor had we acquired any of its jargon. Neither of us had yet come to understand or use the word "conditioning". Kenny, I thought, had a new concept of journalism, a concept as human as the urge she described.

Mary's copy arrived and was published under the title, "Babymania", more dilute than our conversation, still intimate enough to bring a letter or two of protest from women who found her choice of subject "shameful" or "immodest". I tried to get more copy out of her, but I think that she was not impressed by the size of the magazine's cheque.

The next time I heard of Mary Kenny in Dublin was about two years later, when she landed the job of Woman's Editor on the *Irish Press*. Mary, I was told, was sitting in a pub close by on Burgh Quay, waiting for the editor, Tim Pat Coogan, to find an office and furniture for her. Having got the job, she had no intention of beginning on the wrong foot. The *Irish Press* was a warren of overcrowded dingy little offices. Mary, the new executive, was not about to undermine her status by fitting herself obligingly into any old dusty corner. She would not go to work until a proper place was found for her. "Put me on the payroll," she told Tim Pat, "and let me know when you've found an office for me." One was found.

Almost immediately, her Women's Page became so controversial and downright readable that it was often the biggest event of a day. Men read it too. When she got an idea, she could translate it into a whole page in her head with flair and confidence. She had two brilliant young left-wing journalists, Anne Harris and Rosita Sweetman, on her staff. They both tackled sociological subjects in a way that needed doing and had never been done in a woman's page in Ireland before. Rosita Sweetman's first book, *On Our Knees,* was written in the early seventies, and was an excellent attempt to look at contemporary Ireland. I was a free-lance journalist myself by the time Mary came to the *Irish Press,* and I found it great to work for her. She inspired confidence, knew exactly what was wanted and was delighted when it arrived. She seemed to draw female talent out of the woodwork, but she also gave space to the more radical and intellectual people in the community such as Eavan Boland the poet, and Lelia Doolan, the RTE producer who had left that organisation and, with her colleagues Jack Dowling and Bob Quinn had written *Sit Down and Be Counted.*

The Women's Movement followed in the wake of Mary's established Women's Page, and she used the page, as did other women's page editors, to further the cause. Marys Maher and Kenny were undoubtedly the bravest of the editors, but then they did have the most power.

Mary was quite fearless. For instance, when Rosita Sweetman did a London interview with feminist Eva Figes about patriarchal attitudes, she started her piece with: "Now that women masturbate and the whole concept of women's sexuality is being seen in a new way ..." This in a country where masturbation is still called "self-abuse" in the agony columns.

Mary forged ahead; sacred cows mooed anxiously as she attacked. Nor could she be easily suppressed. When eventually Tim Pat Coogan hauled her over the coals for the contents of her page, pointing out her indiscretions and suggesting that she might concentrate on more general subjects for a while, she dispatched a woman reporter to the Dublin Spring Show to write about the prize bull. The Women's Page presented a picture of the noble animal with full discussion of its merits.

The *Irish Times,* under the influence of Mary Maher, an

Irish-American journalist from Chicago, had begun the revolution. Radical talk seemed somehow more natural in that paper. Written largely by socialists and intellectuals, the *Irish Times* reflected its readers' readiness to accept changing concepts. Nor did it sacrifice its "old money" tone. The Social and Personal column painstakingly charted, daily, the whereabouts of the Earl of Here or There, and let its readers know whether the Hon. So-and-So and his Lady were staying in the Shelbourne, the Royal Hibernian or the Russell. Perhaps it was the constant presence of such notable sophisticates which made the *Irish Times* readers less vulnerable to shock. Anyway, hadn't most of them been using contraceptives for years, acquired, no doubt, from the same Georgian square in which I got my little cap?

Apart from all that, Mary Maher was a less flamboyant and more politically circumspect person. Her quieter assurance, a contrast to Mary Kenny's thrusting confidence, represented a different cultural experience. Mary Maher was in college when Betty Friedan's *Feminine Mystique* was launched, and she remembers the class discussing it with their professor of literature. Although Friedan illustrated that the American woman graduate was regressing from emancipation and scurrying into domesticity, still Mary Maher and her peers had got to the point of discussing it. The young American woman expected to achieve, expected to reach goals during her college years. Mary Maher expected to work, to succeed. Mary Kenny, determined to do both, appeared to be merely doing what came naturally, but she must constantly have had to remind herself, in the context of Irish society, that it was not a fantasy she was living but real life. Certainly, in the *Irish Press* she seemed a petunia in a parsnip patch.

The *Irish Press* hung there, like an amazing indestructible cobweb, when Mary came along. Why she approached it at all had a lot to do with the sentimental aspect of the Kenny personality, as well as her ravenous ego. She would shine at home where, still, recognition means most to her. She would be centre stage, her favourite position, in

Dublin, her favourite place. And when the women's movement came along, she assumed the extra rôle of changing the world for women. Perhaps it was then that she began to recognise that the dry and dusty web housed the essence of no less a patriarchy than the Fianna Fáil party.

Why did the *Irish Press* hire Mary Kenny? True, the Women's Movement hadn't come into its own when she arrived. Still, it is hardly likely that her uproarious potential was not recognised. Also, at the time, with all that happened in the sixties, all the changes, all the promises, in media terms it must have seemed like a good idea to give her her head. But I believe it went deeper than that. It was the unconscious thrust of the powers that be towards the possibility for change. Certainly, a man as politically aware and media-minded as Tim Pat Coogan must have been excited by the fresh breezes blowing around Mary Kenny. And it often happens that when change is in the air, even august bodies entertain covert, unconscious fantasies about a new world, only to back off when it looks as though change might actually happen. It took no time at all before splutterings were heard from the Burgh Quay establishment. Not that she was aware of what was happening. She took her ongoing tussles with Tim Pat as part of their excellent relationship.

"They had been so nice to me," she says now, "and it was a bit mean of me really, but I plunged ahead with the zealousness of youth." She recalls picking her way up the rickety stairs of the *Irish Press* wearing a leather mini-skirt, carrying a placard demanding:"Free Contraceptives Now".

There was the paper, unofficial organ of the government, trying to contain this incredible embarrassment, an embarrassment presumably shared by many voters, for the subsequent coalition government did not come any nearer to solving the problem of family planning. Along with the embarrassment, of course, Mary was the source of much vicarious delight. An old colleague, says Mary, went to see her in London recently and she opened the door, very tired, her hair all over the place, in some old smock, the baby's bottle in her hand. He looked at her and said: "To

119

think I used to have sex fantasies about you."

She had this ability to excite, to arouse people's fantasies, sexual or otherwise. Her energy, through the media, turned people on to all sorts of possibilities. There are those who would argue about Mary Kenny's importance to the Irish Women's Movement, some doubting that she was ever genuinely committed at all to anything but her own place in the limelight, her own career. Certainly, there were those committed who made less personal gain. Mary was the big turn-on, though. She was much criticised among our group for accepting the rôle of spokeswoman every chance she got. In those days, few women were called to the cause, fewer were chosen. Mary chose to be at the forefront and was recognised by the public as the One. Whether as a sister or as an enemy of "femininity" — God, what a valuable commodity that suddenly became — she accepted the rôle utterly unconscious of possible consequences.

As a conscious feminist, although she had not yet had a chance to integrate that consciousness, Mary was a rebellious media opportunist, the obvious *enfant terrible* through whose lips the sad, angry and secret thoughts of Irish women could be expressed. She spoke for women who never found their own true voices — until the time when she began to question her first thoughts, and then many broke silence to eat Mary alive.

In the Ireland of the early seventies, when Kenny was in her heyday, she represented the new woman. She was part of the changing energy in the world. She was blatantly a cosmopolitan lass, reminding us of the enormous energy in the world of the 'sixties. Surely everyone was touched by that international energy, the thrust towards human potential. Kenny, more than anyone else, it seemed, was vibrant with this potential. She was grasped by the public in their effort to unite with that energy. And, of course, that union was never consummated, for as the aspirations swelled like balloons, soaring out of the obvious reach of so many, people ran scared, retreated into "reality". Defensive mutterings became progressively more extreme.

"Ah come now." "This is going too far." "Unfeminine."
"Lesbians." "Harlots, threatening the family." "A disgrace
to Irish womanhood." None of us had ever been allowed
to explore what Irish womanhood might be, but now we
threatened it. It was apparently something terribly
precious, something to be protected at all costs — or more
accurately, at any cost at all to the women concerned.
Equal pay would affect our womanhood, birth control
would affect our womanhood, and so there was the sound
of rhubarb across the land. Even those who believed they
wanted change were terrified when they heard the din of
shells cracking for the omelette. I have experienced this
feeling so often myself. Changes change people, and it is
hard to pay the price of becoming a different person when
the old person must inevitably tag along.

> Because the mass, and ourselves as part of that mass,
> are reluctant to start the journey, those who do are
> made, at best, scapegoats and, at worst, victims. The
> public issues are neatly converted into the "mad
> person" and the remainder can hold the picture of
> being "civilised" and "contented". The impotence is
> locked away.
>
> (W. Gordon Lawrence,
> "The Management of Oneself in Role").

Did any two sentences ever better describe what happened
to Mary Kenny and the other mouths of the movement?
What better explains the right wing, conservative backlash
against all world peoples' revolution, which comes in waves
as predictable as the sea? Perhaps those who are most
aware of the danger of uncovering their own pain bleat the
loudest, protesting against subjectivity on the part of the
articulate, proclaiming their own "normality". Normality,
in the context of women's lives, is just another word for
the devil you know, patriarchy, being better than the devil
you've never tried, autonomy. To protect one from the
agony of gaining autonomy there must be an acceptance of
the "natural order" of things. Voicelessness. Silent screams.

Not that the Irish Women's Liberation Movement was anything like as fierce or effective as the American one, for all our marching, demonstrating and talking. But in the early 'seventies, I have no doubt, we were enough for Ireland to be getting on with. I remember the time Mary paused with a doughy sandwich roll en route to her mouth and said: "Y'know, somebody who knows a lot about such things tells me Women's Liberation will never catch on in Ireland. Maybe they're right. Still, it's fun, isn't it? And it *feels* as if something is happening."

Her energy knew no bounds. She could stay up most of the night partying and drinking and she'd be up and on the 'phone arranging stories and talking to her bank manager before anyone else was ready for her. Then she'd paint the face. Mary's face was always painted rather than made up. She believed paint was fun. When it became a necessity or a disguise it entered into the realm of neurosis. And no matter what the hurry, before she dressed she would try on outfit after outfit, appraising herself in the mirror. Never anything as dull as smart clothes. But she had piles of tat, combinations that looked zany, even shabby, since they had been hauled out of a trunk at "Gainsborough" or London's Portobello Road rag shops. They looked Kennyish. She enjoyed our enjoyment of them. And of course, there were her long-stemmed velvet pipes.

I know these early morning details because Nell McCafferty, then a reporter with the *Irish Times*, was close friends with Kenny. Being with Mary was like being at a party all the time, Nell used to say. When she stayed over at the Kenny flat, Mary would be up with the lark. Then while she did her telephoning and organised her page, she'd prepare a four-course breakfast for her pal. She didn't eat breakfast, but carried in the silver tray, the lot, complete with rose. And she'd clear it away before she left for work with: "You were born to lie in bed, darling, but I really must be off."

Mary's gaiety did not distract from her competence in the slightest and if it irritated those who seemed drearily obsessed with being grey and working-class in those days, she remained irrepressible. She learned from everyone with whom she spent time: politicians, government ministers, businessmen and the literary types who lived in Dublin's pubs. She threw parties, rumours of which made one jealous not to have received an invitation.

"Did you really have drugs and group sex at those parties?" I asked.

"Well, we had lots of drink and ciggies, but I don't think group sex. Not really. Actually, we did take our clothes off, but everybody looked sort of white and cold and nonchalant and it didn't work. I didn't ask you because I thought you'd disapprove," she flashed. "I mean you had children and all." Then I remembered having brought her home for a meal one night with my children. She was a delightful, interested and relaxed guest. "That sort of thing is such a lovely change, thank you," she said. I think I had forgotten to serve wine with the meal.

Sometimes she would have a really dangerous idea. I remember one which, fortunately, came to nothing. Half a dozen free-lancers were having lunch on the floor in Mary's office, and she hit on the idea of experimenting with swapping life-styles. I, she thought, would be ideal to go out to Ballymun high-rise flats and take over some woman's husband and children while she moved into my home in Rathfarnham and lived the life of a divorcée with three children. The idea was a grabber, but terrifying. It became more dicey as it was teased out. Still, Mary thought it would make a brilliant page, or even two, in the *Irish Press;* a high rise flat with small kids and me as a housewife with a husband coming into his tea at six o'clock. Oh God, I thought on the way home, don't let Mary find anyone to swap lives with me. I need not have worried. Tim Pat promptly shot the idea down. Mary could understand his apprehension, but she felt he had behaved a bit bossily. Still, she would diary the idea for the future. Has that time yet arrived? Not for me with yer man in Ballymun, anyway.

Maher and Kenny must have done most of the recruitment to the original women's group, so it wasn't surprising there were so many journalists among us. I remember sitting beside Kenny in the room over Gaj's restaurant where we met in those days. I asked her, "Who is that?" "That," she grinned, looking at Nuala Fennell, "is my link with suburbia, and those women with her must be the Toni twins." They were Maura Humphreys and Bernadette Quinn, sisters, and her remark was about their neat hairstyles.

From the start, Mary could not be hushed. It was agreed that anyone could speak in her own right but not as spokesperson for everybody, but, too often, it didn't happen like that with Kenny. Also, she often assumed inappropriate authority. I remember being terribly hurt by her, one Saturday evening, having worked for days with Mary Earls photostatting and stapling together our booklet "Chains or Change". In breezed Kenny, blowing smoke and smelling of champagne, and thanked me graciously as if I were a parlour maid who had just handed her a tray. "I didn't do it for *you*," I said pettily, "we're all doing our bit." "But of course, how thoughtless of me," she replied.

"The greatest enemy of women's liberation is women," Mary raged at a meeting in 1970. "Our bitterest criticism comes from women." Women would not, she said, elect other women to the Dáil and they would attempt to tear down any other female who was not an obedient conformist to the male vision of things. The reason for this was not because women were naturally jealous — there was no evidence that they were any more jealous than men — but the much more troubling one that women were full of self-hate. Therefore, they had no confidence in other women.

She declared that women's self-hate was the reason they wore cosmetics, in an effort to camouflage their true selves. Irish women did not want to be liberated and were insulted by the very suggestion. They preferred to rely on the protection of men, settling for a seat on the bus instead of their adult rights. Irish women insisted on being girly girls who acted out the rules that male society had designed for them.

It is strange to realise, looking back, that Mary was only

with us for two years. Then, out of the blue, came her big London chance. The editor of the *Evening Standard* rang her and asked her to come and have lunch with him in the Savoy Hotel. "And, of course, I loved the idea of flying to London for lunch and it was a very, very nice lunch. I love London. It had been so exciting when I was living there in the swinging sixties. And then he said 'Will you come to London as features editor?' and I said I would think about it. I was thrilled to be offered this job, y'know."

Mary was twenty-seven years old and would be the youngest executive ever employed by the paper, as well as the only woman executive. They offered her £1,800, a lot of money in those days. She cried all the way back on the 'plane because of the conflict involved. Here was a fork in her life. In some ways she felt she ought to stay in Ireland, but she felt she owed it to herself to take this opportunity. "I had this wild fear that if I didn't go back to Fleet Street now I'd never be asked again. It was a purely careerist decision."

At home she dithered for a while. The atmosphere in the *Irish Press*, Rosita Sweetman recalls, was like that in a family with a divorce pending. Tim Pat Coogan was furious. Handful that she was, he had backed her up and he felt she was being selfish.

After she went, the Women's Page regressed. Compared to what it had been, it became as soggy as a baby's diaper and has never regained the wild unpredictability of Mary's day.

Across the water, Mary's first year on the *Evening Standard* as Features Editor was sheer misery. She was lonely, and had a sense of having run out on us. Apart from that, she says now, she wasn't up to the job. She didn't have the experience, but more especially the confidence, since many of her staff were older men and didn't seem to know what she was about. It was a different mood, anyway. The swinging 'sixties were over, Northern Ireland was the great problem and Mary, naturally, was a very Republican girl.

"I kept saying 'we have to do something about Northern

Ireland'." In 1972, the *Evening Standard* had a very strong philosophy that Ireland simply wasn't important. After all, it's a London, not national paper, read by the Queen. "I was very agitated about this going on, you know, and I couldn't let up. I remember saying again we should do something about Ireland in conference one day and one of my mates said 'Mary, for God's sake stop about Ireland. You'll never be a good London journalist until you put that bloody country out of your head'."

About a year after she got the job she gave it up and became European correspondent of the *Evening Standard* instead. It didn't help her sense of exile from Ireland and the Women's Movement. Now she lived a gypsy life, moving around from one European country to another. She describes it as being hell on earth. In 1973 she was sitting in a bar in Frankfurt, feeling like death, with the whole week-end ahead of her. She remembers thinking: "What the hell am I doing with the Common Market anyway, it's meaningless, it's ridiculous, it's completely irrelevant to my life. What do I care about the Common Agricultural Policy, or some other distant boring, unimportant thing? The next morning I sort of wandered around the city and went into a church and sat down. And I thought that's what I really need, just a bit of peace and quiet and reflection. It was just very peaceful and nice. So every now and then in Frankfurt or Brussels or Milan I would go into a church and sit down. I didn't get religion all of a sudden. Nothing like that. You tend to turn to the Church when you are very low. I don't think that anyone would dispute that. It was pleasant to sit in a still, quiet place."

Not that Mary quickly developed stillness or quietness. There was still plenty of fire in the belly. From Rome, about then, she wrote one of her strongest pieces ever, defending the women's movement in reply to criticism of it in the *Sunday Press.* Mary attacked the idea that some beautiful or talented women can do quite nicely in a man's world: "But your special position depends upon your keeping your sisters down. You can't go through life thinking how well *you've* made out, you clever little girl."

Her article concluded: "And already the movement has started having its effects, not just in legislation and job trends, but in human dignity. All over the world, because of it, more women are beginning to hold their heads up a little more, have a little more genuine respect for themselves in the fullest sense, consider themselves as persons, human beings, first class citizens and not any more just sexual objects whose job is to titillate, cajole, provide pleasure and generally accessorise a man's existence. Don't knock it!"

Obviously at this stage, slipping into churches for a bit of peace, Mary still saw herself as a committed champion of feminism. In *Woman X Two,* the book published in 1978 which tried to show the working mother how to cope with a double life, she looked back on the women's movement. "Ruthless social change had to be pursued so that conditions could be created in which men and women were completely and utterly different in every way; if necessary, we would have to rebuild society brick by brick, until that was achieved. It might hurt a few people, but you couldn't make an omelette without breaking eggs."

But things had changed for Mary before she wrote those words. We'd heard that she was getting married to Dick West. Patrick, their son, was born. The baby changed her life, her perception of what her life must be, claims Mary. Certainly, the infant appears to have ousted the fire in Mary's belly. She was overwhelmed by maternal awareness. Then along came Edward, her second son. Now she became the prodigal daughter. Her musings about domesticity were intertwined with religious fervour and an inevitably self-righteous undertone. A born-again Christian? Those at home hooted. But it was to get worse. Now it seemed that everything she wrote was from the pulpit. She had been a wicked foolish girl, she confessed with boring regularity in print, on air and on television. If only she had not been so irresponsible.

In 1979 I did a face-to-face interview with her for an Irish magazine. It was in the form of question and answer and I tried to get answers for all the questions which people were asking about the new Mary Kenny. During the course of the interview she told me she had had an abortion in the early 'seventies. I left it out of the copy, but had to ring the editor to include it when I heard Kenny announce the fact to the Irish nation on the radio a day after my copy was delivered. She was a Christian and she must bear witness, she told me. No, she didn't use contraceptives, but her husband did. Yes, he was a male chauvinist, but who could teach an old dog new tricks? Dick West was her best friend, had developed her intellectually, gave her books to read, talked to her. She wasn't a great mother, she feared, her children were always covered in chocolate, etc. etc. She had a Jungian tutor. RTE radio used the article as the basis of at least two programmes about Mary Kenny and feminism.

The last time I met Mary, she had finished her book, *Why Christianity Works.* She was in a post partum state of depression. Well, she said, after all the research, all the work, it was bound to be superficial, wasn't it? What book on such an enormous subject wouldn't be, except the New Testament? Yet her ambition had driven her "forward" once again.

"Are you happy that Christianity works?" I asked.

"No, I'm not. I think one has only to look at the Spanish Inquisition and wonder where it all went wrong. I don't think it works as a social theory or anything like that, but I think it can work as a personal system. But it is not really justified, Christianity, although it has to be my witness, so therefore it's basically about Roman Catholicism. The book is more defensive of religion, not just Catholicism. It's a repudiation of the Marxist idea that religion is just something forced as a superstructure on people, that it's social conditioning or whatever. It is simply arguing that religion and the moral codes which are parallel and part of religion are fundamental, that they are archetypal in the way they are stamped on us, in the way that 'Brighton Rock' is stamped through Brighton rock."

"Could you possibly talk about your relationship with

Christ?" I asked her.

"Well, I don't know how well that's developed, actually."

"But if you don't have feelings about Christ, what's the sense of bothering yourself with Christianity at all? I mean, it's just my opinion. But if Christ isn't the centre of your Christianity, well, you're kind of having a love affair without a lover?"

"Well yes, I think Christ is at the centre of one's Christianity, but at the same time one cannot say that anyone who is not a Christian is lost." Later she says: "I think that the exploration of the meaning of life grows very much out of the Women's Movement experience. When I was reading the story of Martin Luther, *Matter of Human Aggression,* I remember sitting on a Number 11 bus and I wanted to dig the woman in front of me and say: 'you've got to read this, it is so fantastic.' It reminded me so much of the women's movement, the constant revolution, the awakening of the individual spirit, the finding of a voice to rebel against the clergy class, rebelling against a hierarchy which said: 'We don't have a God for you and we won't tell you.' It was suddenly the individual awakening and saying 'We won't accept the priestly caste, we won't accept the corruption and all the carry-on.' It's impossible not to be on the side of Martin Luther. It reminded me of the women's movement because of the developing consciousness and it also reminded me of the women's movement because in throwing off one tyranny, Luther took on another. He threw off the tyranny of the princes and the cardinals and priests and so on and he took on, in a way, the tyranny of himself and suffered the pain and the guilt. Also, it was very interesting in terms of masculine and feminine as well, because Luther rebelled, he had this ambiguous relationship with God. He wanted to throw off the authority of God which was pressing down on him all the time. As soon as he threw off the authority of God, he felt much greater guilt. I think women feel that about men."

"I don't. A man is not God. The freer I become, the more autonomous, the less guilty I feel. It doesn't make me feel guilty not to be bossed."

"Yes, but what I am saying is that no revolution ever just alters the orthodoxy, it replaces it with another orthodoxy."

I asked her to come back to her own experience.

"I think I went into the movement irresponsibly. I mean, I felt rebellious against the way things were in Ireland. But it was an involvement which made me think, really think, about the meaning of life and about the individual and about why we do certain things, who we are ..."

"Who are you, Mary?"

"Well, an old friend saw me recently after a long time and she said: 'I'm either going to punch you in the face or kiss you.' And I said: 'You'll have to make up your own mind,' and she kissed me and said: 'Mary, for a handful of gold you left us.' That was painful. Where's the handful of gold? In fact if I had my life over again in the last ten years, if I had realised what I would go through in being very public about my feelings, I think I would have held my tongue. I would just quietly have done what so many people have done, what I see so many women do, carrying on the orthodoxies of their peers and just quietly changing their lives. All the friends that I knew in London in the 'sixties, who were very left-wing and so on, I see them just quietly sending their children to private schools and quietly moving into the easy capitalist way of life, going on writing neutral things that they don't have to commit themselves to and just sort of quietly changing their lines about things. All the women who said life had to be absolutely free and then digging their ex-husbands for all the alimony they could get, accepting the system. I should have been prudent about it really. I should have thought things through."

In the autumn of 1979 Kenny, the newspaper woman par excellence, was finding that some of her old newspaper contacts had turned against her. She felt down about that. "You know that in journalism so much is done by connections. Of course, I've attacked *Cosmopolitan* magazine, for instance, so it isn't surprising."

I come to her defence: "But magazines like Cosmo are sinister in their effect on young women. Imagine being an ordinary young woman, with an ordinary job, ordinary assets, and you look at Cosmo and you're supposed to have money in the bank and you're supposed to be a brain surgeon, a sexy brain surgeon and you're supposed to be having an abortion on your afternoon off. I mean, would you not feel there was something wrong with you, that you had failed somehow?"

"Yes, and the most awful thing about the magazine is that the typical Cosmopolitan reader is a young woman in her early twenties, living in Birmingham with two small children in a high-rise block. But at the same time, Deirdre McSharry is not cynical ... Anyway even my original mentor in British journalism won't hire me anymore. He said: 'Mary was such fun when she was into sex, but now she's into religion and she's such a bore', and so I don't fit in here or there."

"What now?" I feel vaguely ashamed on behalf of everybody.

"I'm more supportive of the Women's Movement now than I was two years ago. I think I'm through all the violent change that was going through my life. Not having confidence in oneself, that's so hard, June. I've been so lonely. I absolutely understand why human beings are so conformist. Now I understand why people did not stand up to the Third Reich, or whatever, because it is so hard to be different, to lose friends. The most awful thing that happened to me was in County Clare where we took the children for a holiday a couple of years ago. Dick was working and I was alone most of the month. I hate the country. It think it is so philistine and boring, there are no book shops and no theatre and no one to talk to. It's frightfully dreary and I couldn't get to a pub because of the kids. Then someone told me there was a writer's workshop on locally and I went and nobody would talk to me except Proinnsias MacAonghusa and I love him forever."

"Who was there?"

"Donal Foley and all the old gang. I spent a lot of time sitting by myself. And I went over to an old friend and she said: 'Mary, I really don't want to talk to you.' She wouldn't talk to me. It was such a blow to my self-esteem and made me feel so nervous."

"But you hurt a lot of people, being so noisy about turning tail, Mary. It felt like a betrayal. I was raging with you for a while. Thought you were never going to shut up."

"I understand. Of course I do, intellectually. It must have seemed to people as if I was shitting on them." I look up startled by her uncharacteristic language. Her face is very white. "But I feel too, why can't you understand what I am trying to say?"

"What are you trying to say? What would you say to women who point out that when it suited you to burn your bra and throw up your knickers, you did that, and that now when the women that were tied down by babies at the time have a chance to start living their own lives a bit, you're telling them there was a mistake. I mean, what do you say to women who thought Mary Kenny was leading the way?"

"But there weren't supposed to be leaders. The ideology was that each one worked out her own truth. I'm trying to say that life is more complicated than it looks on the surface, that revolutions, great changes, social ideas and people's feelings are much more complicated than they look."

"Who disagrees with that?" I ask.

"Well specifically, the battle for birth control is fundamental in this country and I support it. But I also think that birth control and abortion can and are being used against women just as much. What irritates me is that when Germaine Greer says it, it will be accepted and suddenly people will say oh goodness, Greer shows you that international capitalism exploits women."

"Maybe it is the way you are saying it. And it's not just capitalism. You can't say that an anti-child society is good, but you can't say over-population is good either, and what about women forced into being baby machines?"

"But that is also more complicated than it appears ..."

Crabbily, I recall women pregnant every year, wrecked and broken, but resist the temptation to remind her just how complicated life can be for such a woman and her family.

Nowadays, Mary believes that any pursuit of happiness is selfish. However, she admits that she would like her life to go on as it is with some improvements. She'd like another child passionately, and seems very angry that her husband claims a say in this decision. I find it odd that a fertile young woman finds this such a difficult problem to solve.

She'd like to be working busily, perhaps editing a sort of "Christian Cosmopolitan". She hasn't quite thought that one out. She would also love to be back in Bowe's pub opposite the *Irish Times* with Nell McCafferty, Mary Cummins, Mary Maher and the old gang.

"Accepted as maybe quirky or unpredictable or something, but accepted ... I haven't meant to be malicious, you know."

Currently, Mary Kenny is working on a book about the experience of abortion.

8
IN THE BEGINNING

On a summer's night in 1970, in a large room over Gaj's restaurant in Dublin's Baggot Street, I was quite suddenly aware of being in the right place. I remember being surprised because this meant that I must have felt misplaced for so long without knowing it. Now I belonged. A good feeling came with that, or rather, the merest promise of a feeling, which would develop over the years so that at last I could call it self-acceptance. Even then, I recognised: "I've survived, I'm surviving now. This is surviving." I was thinking about this in one of my mini-trances when a scene came into my head: I was washed ashore, resting on the sand, the sea safely behind me, sun warming my back. I let out a deep sigh of relief and Mary Anderson sitting beside me, asked: "What are you grinning about?"

By the time I had formed an answer for her she was talking to somebody else. It was often like that at meetings of the Irish Women's Liberation Movement. Everybody talked at the same time — not much in the way of manners — but one had the sense of being properly heard for the first time ever, just the same. I looked around the room full of women whom I had known for such a short time, and explored my sense of arrival. Why hadn't I seen it before? These were my people. Not Jews, not Christians. Women. I felt it amazing that somehow I had found my way to this place. As Mary jabbered on, I sat enjoying *myself,* resting on the sand, the ache ebbing from my bones, throat relaxed, touched by faith. It was almost like falling in love.

That was certainly not the first meeting of the founding members of the group. There might have been a dozen meetings before then, but I remember that one best, because of that realisation. Its essence was in the joy of discovering oneself among the others. Other female selves.

Looking back, it seems to me now it was in that room that I first looked into an undistorted mirror of femininity. I got to know some of the women very well, others not at all. Sometimes we fought. And yet the bonding grew. The bonding survived because meeting one of those women after ages makes no difference to the warmth which surfaces, and sisterhood is never further away than the other end of a telephone line.

In 1970, survival was my trip. It crowded my consciousness. I was driven by it. It was like being blind-folded for a long journey, not having a clue as to the destination, but bound to make it. I had escape routes from my frenzied survival trip, work, sex, clothes, tablets and unpinpointed rage. I regarded night as a railway station in which, like a train, I refuelled before continuing. So I often stayed awake, relaxed in the knowledge that the world slept. In the land of Night I could simply be. I could write or read or bake, dare to think without worrying. The battle continued by day.

Survival is always an existential struggle. We may all be in the same leaky boat with the same sharks surrounding us, but each woman's struggle is uniquely hers, driven by its own fuel, coloured by its own consciousness. The loneliness of that had hit me by the time I met that group of women. The wonder revealed by the group was that there was no need for the boat to be leaky; the sharks were made powerful by our passivity. We lived in occupied country. The whole world, for women, was occupied country. We were simply allowed to share what "they" had taken as their own.

Consciousness boiled up from the depths of all the female energy in that room over Gaj's. It uncovered the everyday wounds which we had experienced as females, experienced in isolation, not understanding that it was not all inevitable, discovering that each one of us was not the odd-ball, the only one who could not accept the way things were supposed to be. We discovered that most of us had been damaged, enraged, humiliated by similar things, had felt put down by "normality". In pooling our experiences of life we discovered the world as it was for females. It was not the way it need be. As this consciousness rose I, for one, felt a growing release as if from the weight of a secret I need no longer contain.

I also discovered a strength which came with the ability to identify the source of my anger, and experienced a sense of re-possession of myself as if I were regaining something which had been stolen from me. I could see now that marriage had created an isolation cell for me, divided me from my self, divided me from my own sex. I had been in solitary confinement.

Years later I was to recognise that pre-women's movement state for what it was — emotional and intellectual Purdah. In India, donning Burkha, the Muslim Purdah, I travelled about for a day wrapped up as a man's possession, like a parcel, and wound up feeling the same misery that had been my veiled lot before 1970. Purdah separated me from men, from women — even other women in Purdah — and above all from my whole self. Before Gaj's I had talked to women, listened to them, but what had I said and what had I heard with Purdah separating us? As girls, we had moved towards marriage like lemmings, nudging each other out of the way, the quicker to be the one submerged. The one who won the race threw the bouquet. Sometimes, it was alright to hand the bouquet to the oldest girl yet unmarried. Her need was recognised as greater, and nobody minded ...

It was Mary Kenny who invited me to my first meeting of IWLM. "It's about women's liberation," said Mary, "and it's in Mary Maher's house because she can't get a baby-sitter."

"Liberation from what?" I'd asked her and she gave me a funny look. Mary Maher, the Chicago journalist working on the *Irish Times* had married Des Geraghty, the trade union official and they lived in Strandville Avenue, North Strand, near a railway bridge. I remember wondering as I entered Mary's house why anyone would choose to live in such a dreary street without a garden. I'd lived in a similar street, Lennox Place, off Dolphin's Barn near the canal, when I was a child, but we'd got out of it as quickly as we could to a place with gardens. Mary's house typified my puzzlement with socialists in those days. They always seemed to want to live in working-class streets, in artisan dwelling houses minus a bit of greenery, to wear dreary clothes and affect a certain pennilessness. It was to take some time before I realised that while I blew my money on the bright material things of life now, they were sensibly saving for the future.

I'd barely met Mary Maher, but knew she was a barrister's daughter. She was one of the first with whom the late Donal Foley, news-editor of the *Irish Times* broke the stereotype of women's journalism in Ireland. She was doing the same work as a male journalist. Máirin de Burca, then an official of Sinn Féin, had brought along two American feminists. Dr. Máire Woods, now of Dublin's Well Woman Centre, was deeply involved in left-wing politics, as was Margaret Gaj, a Scottish woman married to a Pole whose restaurant in Baggot Street was a centre of radicals during the 'sixties and part of the 'seventies. To visit her restaurant was an experience in meeting people who were fired up about everything from corporal punishment in schools to housing or nuclear development. Men or women, the people who ate at Gaj's had an earnest air about them.

There was Máirin Johnston, who was an activist with the Labour Party, later a member of the Communist Party, an ardent trade unionist whose main interest nowadays is the development of pre-school facilities.

There was Mary Sheerin, recently returned from working in Paris, a secretary with the National Publishing Company at the time, now with Government Information and a published short-story writer. Mary was my close friend, a younger woman of amazing sophistication in the broadest sense of the word, sensitive and *sympathique*, a devout Catholic with strong family attachments. She had, early in life, as one of a family of five girls, registered injustice to women, but even in relation to this she had a marvellous sense of humour.

Mary McCutchan, women's editor of the *Irish Independent*, was there, a meticulous workaholic who nonetheless seemed to move in an unflurried aura of being in love. She was engaged to the man she married, Eamonn Fingleton, a journalist, now in London's Fleet Street. Mary was killed in the mid-seventies in a London traffic accident with her six-week-old twins.

Mary Anderson, also of the *Irish Independent* woman's page, with her mop of black curls, was to become for a while the angriest and most alarming voice of the movement. Her energy matched her anger and often, when she spoke, it seemed as if all female rage was channelling itself through her. She had a love-hate relationship with journalism which she left, first to study Politics at Ruskin College, Oxford and then finally to join an alternative life-styles ranch in the US, to which she had got a scholarship to study drama. She was a natural actress with a lovely singing voice.

Then, of course, there was Nuala Fennell, now a TD in Dáil Éireann, then a housewife breaking into free-lance journalism.

There was a lot of heavy talk at that meeting in Mary Maher's; it was decided to launch a women's movement in Ireland. It all seemed a bit unreal to me. We seemed to be discussing a small matter of changing the world. The American voices rose above the others, although I remember that our answers to their questions startled me more than the questions themselves. God, things were humiliating for Irish women. The status of women in Ireland was a depressing area for examination. I remember feeling ashamed in front of the Americans, humiliated by the Irish condition of womanhood, but I could see the visitors didn't see their own lot as that much better than ours. I'd been shocked myself, upon returning home from Canada, at the obviously lower standard of living here, but we talked about things that went deeper than that. The status of a woman in a family or in a nation has little to do with the standard of living. Comfort is not freedom. In any case, these Americans didn't brag about what they had back home. Even then, international feminism was largely free of chauvinist pride in relation to female status. We were all women in the same world. It was heavy going, though. So much talk, talk that raised cringing feelings long since buried. I was delighted when Mary Maher's infant daughter woke up and I got hold of her.

"Have you all that to look forward to, little woman?" I asked the child, cuddling her as much for my own sake as hers. Later Nell McCafferty arrived. Always late.

"What have yez been talking about?" she asked in her dead-pan Derry drawl, innocent of the fact that we'd have our work cut out summing up that lot for her. I can't remember whether it was that night at Mary Maher's or another time in Mary Kenny's flat that there was the business of the cheese. From the beginning it had been decided that any attempt at "middle-class hostessing" was out. No baking. No serving anything but coffee. We were liberating ourselves from all that. This cheese board was carried in and placed with the mugs. A serious discussion developed about "entertaining" and offering cheese boards. One of the two Marys — yes, it was Kenny — promised that she would never transgress again. Every scrap of the cheese was devoured.

That group of 'seventies feminists began in Bewley's of Westmoreland Street, Dublin. The five women present were all involved in left-wing radical activities of the 'sixties: Margaret Gaj, Mary Maher, Máirin Johnston, Máire Woods and Máirin de Burca. They had met a few times before the rest of us joined them in Mary Maher's house that night. Obviously, it was a set-up. Kenny had invited as middle-class a bunch as she could lay hands on, and would continue to do so for a while. How the original five must have blinked when they saw the rest of us arrive. So we began with that split. It more or less lasted, but with the interesting, if hardly unexpected development that like a marriage of co-operative opposites, each side learned from the other. Eventually, there would be feminist socialists and socialist feminists and of course the small number of women who moved not an inch from their original position. Altogether, the group came to sixteen or so, with a few women on the fringe dropping in or around, sometimes dropping out after a few meetings.

One of the most active women in the group was a young woman whose long blond hair often hid what she was thinking in a discussion. Marie McMahon was the first female printer I had ever met. She was a friend of the Gaj family and a true political child of the 'sixties. Her concern for humans spilled over to animals to such an extent that when she gave me one of her pet's puppies she paid "public health" nursing visits to my home regularly until she was sure the puppy, now an old lady, was being responsibly reared.

Fionnuala O'Connor, a school teacher from Lisburn, was unemployed when I met her first. A keenly intelligent woman, she was also politically active and a born writer. Eventually, she got a job on the *Irish Times,* went to work for them in Belfast and is these days heard of as being "blissfully married" with a family and still the *Irish Times* person in Belfast.

Eavan Boland, the poet, was a founder member who wrote literary pieces for Mary Kenny's woman's page. Tall, slim, the English Rose type, Eavan looked nothing like the other Irish poets of the 'sixties. She was neither dishevelled or malnourished in appearance, giving away the fact that she probably managed to write her poems without the support of Dublin's literary pub culture.

Dr. Eimer Philbin Bowman was another. A quiet young woman, she was a doctor with an academic air and two small children. She was trying to work out a balance in her life at the time between career and motherhood. Having been reared by a professional woman, her own mother, she was later to tell me that it came as a surprise to her that it was difficult to have two rôles. "It hadn't dawned on me that working as a mother could be difficult because my mother always worked. She still works and babysits for me!"

Bernadette Quinn was a pharmacist, married to a pharmacist, who came along with her sister Rosemary Humphries. Bernadette declared that they had been reared equally with their brothers and yet her short stories, one of which won The Maxwell House Short Story Competition for women, clearly revealed that she knew the ground which bred feminism. She was also co-author, with Nuala Fennell and Deirdre McDevitt of *Can You Stay Married?* Rosemary, child-rearing full time, has since returned to nursing.

The independent-minded Hilary Boyle, who worked as a journalist specialising in radio talks and articles on nature and gardening, assured us that she had led a liberated life. She lived in a tiny room not much larger than a decent closet in Pembroke Road and seemed involved in everything. She was obsessed with the problem of contraception in a way atypical of an elderly woman and she believed in the women's movement as a source of help for poor women. She used a stick to walk, but she could out-march and out-demonstrate any of us, and did. She departed the group because we would not invite men to join us.

Mary Earls was an energetic member. She always seemed to have read the latest book first, so it wasn't a surprise when upon marrying Don Roberts, a fellow left-winger, she moved to Kilkenny where together they set up a thriving book-shop. Later, they moved into second-hand book-selling, and now with three children they have branched out into their own publishing business.

There were the Sweetman girls, Rosita and Inez. Rosita was author of *On Our Knees* about Dublin in the 'sixties, and *Fathers Come First,* a book about growing up in an Irish convent. *On Our Backs*, later, was about Irish sexual attitudes. Rosita was stirred up, early on, about what she described as the anti-male thing, the blaming of men for everything. In fact, what she was aware of was the necessity to locate one's own misery, one's own responsibility in it, and she felt that too many women simply walloped men.

Although the women's movement was well underway in the United States by then, Betty Friedan having founded the National Organisation for Women (NOW) to campaign for equal rights and opportunities in 1966, we in Dublin were all pretty vague about how those equal rights and opportunities could be defined for Irish women. There were groups in London since '68 and '69. Still, the strange stirring, the sense of dissatisfaction or yearning described by Friedan in 1963 when I was staggering blindly through my life, hadn't publicly surfaced in Ireland. The women in that room over Gaj's — and I always think of us as the Gaj's group — weren't at all sure of what we wanted. It certainly was not more of the same.

A great deal of pain surfaced in that room, anger and frustration so symptomatic of our culture that it was often difficult to seek out the origin. I often tried to disown some of the realisations that came into focus, even as I recognised the attempts of others to disown bits of the female experience too painful to be applicable to the self. My own trick was to shrug sometimes. After all, the Catholic Church hadn't got me, had it? I'd been able to get contraception from the beginning. I'd got a divorce, hadn't I?

In delving into our experiences, throwing up personal revelations that were shared by so many, it became all too easy to externalise one's problems. One became a victim of the political system, a system which must be changed to facilitate women, but who would work on changing the self? Change changes people and some of us were to confess to having the same old misery lurking around inside ourselves after more external change than we had ever imagined possible had come to pass. Not that we were only into misery. We discovered humour and, cruelly, satire.

I believe it was more difficult for the women like myself who were or had been married, had children, had been otherwise engaged while the marches, the demonstrations, the struggles to liberate the blacks, the Red Indians and the anti-Vietnam thing had been going on. None of that had much to do with me, had impinged if at all from a distance. I'd been in a rôle. As a middle-class wife in Canada I had done voluntary work, the spare-time hobby expected of me, but politics? And yet, by association, we all contributed to the loosening of each other's shackles. The energy of those meetings, the sheer exhilaration was incredible. Exhausted, I often staggered out, down the stairs and yet totally refreshed. In between meetings, unless something was planned, I led another life with other people, other women who were unconscious, unbothered, uninterested. And it was always great to get back to Gaj's.

With such a diverse collection of people, it was inevitable that interests varied, priorities differed and disagreements were passionate. Everybody wanted change, but while the socialists wanted the entire fabric of society changed from the bottom up, especially in relation to organisation within the family, alternatives to the nuclear family seemed far-fetched to the rest of us, most of whom favoured piecemeal reforms. The socialists were more interested in action. Mary Kenny and myself were hell bent on consciousness-raising. Often one found oneself torn by both groups, confused by two somewhat blurred ideologies. The socialists seemed experienced in one way; they'd been through political procedures, licked the envelopes for the men and made the coffee, and were sure that after the revolution everything would be different for women. The great thing was that we were all talking a new language. A stumbling language it was, especially in the very early days, but gradually it emerged as the sound of autonomy, the language of personal political power. Of course, women had talked a blue streak about parts of their lives and their families since Eve, but now the secrets came to the surface. We could identify a personal context. We began to draw political conclusions from our personal experiences.

The question most often asked was my old favourite, why? Now the "why" raged. Why were women devalued?

Why were we so abused, undermined, chained to the service of others? Why was no value put on that service? Why were we conned into being put on pedestals, taught to be dependent, treated like slaves? Why did men hate us? If they didn't, then why did they act as if they did? Why did we hate ourselves, distrust ourselves, distrust each other? Why did we believe in our own powerlessness?

A painful part of those meetings was seeing myself as others saw me or as I felt they saw me, a man's woman. For years I had been prattling away about beauty, fashion, things around the house, how to camouflage tiredness when your husband came home weary from his work, how to look well-groomed: "after all, since you are the one who does the ironing there is no excuse for not having all your clothes in pristine condition, ready to wear," I wrote. Now that I no longer had a husband willing to come home at all, I'd dropped the formula-for-wedded-bliss bit, but still continued with the rest. I'd come back from the Paris fashion shows wincing at the sight of Dublin women, saying it only took a little effort to look French.

True, I ran a useful problem page and went to great lengths to get people helpful information, but never, ever, had I equated their problems with anything more realistic than bad luck or their own inadequacy. How could I, since I hadn't done as much for myself? I remember a day late in 1969 when I found an American pamphlet, a women's publication, in a seat in the lounge of the Intercontinental Hotel. I'd spent the morning writing an article about how to look better dressed on less money. Now I read: "Women are an oppressed class ... we are exploited as sex objects, breeders, domestic servants and cheap labour." "You can say that again," I muttered wearily and marked down two more ideas for articles, "Health Diet for Better Looks" and "Look Younger at Any Age". Had I dared be honest I'd have written "look sexier", but sex was synonymous with youth anyway. Women knew what I meant. "Look younger" was simply an acceptable way of saying "look sexier".

Before I came to the Gaj's group, I had left *Irishwoman's*

Journal when it was sold to new owners, and was free-lancing. I had as my office base a desk in Kevin Clear Ltd., Waterloo Road. He was a publisher at the time, to this day my dear friend and the first man in Ireland, I believe, to give "women's lib" house space. This was remarkable of him, considering he had six daughters and didn't quite grasp at the time how it was possible for a houseful of girls to be oppressed. Indeed, his daughters were strong, talented, lively young women. It was from Kevin's office that the IWLM manifesto, *Chains or Change* was first published. Mary Earls and myself fed it off his copying machine during a week of nights and one long Saturday. One of my freelance jobs was helping him to get out a publication guiding people along the Shannon, the experience of which sparked off my love of that beautiful river. "I wish," I once wrote somewhere, "I could be like the River Shannon, so much herself, contained yet free." The sub-editor cut the sentence out of the article. "I didn't know what it meant," he said. I don't think that I quite knew what I meant then either. Now I know that it was the central strength, the vital power of the Shannon claimed from nowhere but herself that struck me. Like the central core of a person, the Shannon runs through Ireland. The Shannon, vaguely obscured in relation to other people, in the widening of the world, reminds me of how the centre of a person can be forgotten even by her or himself in relation to the world. And yet that core, that river vein is the source of all strength.

I was also doing a book on *Irish Beauty.* If you were Irish, this book was aimed at helping you to make the most of your natural good looks. I wrote in the editorial: "The average Irish girl may have vitality and a sense of humour; she tends to lack confidence. This lack of confidence or even shame over the idea of being interested in one's physical attributes often springs from early education ... Then, too, Irish families are usually quite large, with an abundance of teasing brothers willing and ready to highlight a girl's weak points while making heavy demand on her time."

This last was apropos of my sending my daughter off
to school as a weekly boarder in an effort to break my two
boys of the habit of treating her as a mother. The calls of
"Di, do I have socks?" or "Di, what's for supper?" fell
upon my ears once too often. If I had let this happen, I
could stop it. I could now recognise those sounds for what
they were, the cannibalistic calls of males. Weren't we
always describing that in the group? Girls doing menial
work, taking responsibility for brothers' comfort. It is, I
learned, easier to cure males of the expectation of being
served than it is to break the habit of serving.

Confidence, I confidently wrote, "is gained by knowing
one is doing one's best on all fronts and this annual deals
with an important aspect of femininity — good grooming ...
your appearance isn't a major issue in life, but it con-
tributes to your sense of well-being which is important ... a
woman enjoys looking as well as she can, so why not be
organised about it?"

I had decided that beauty mainly depended on basic
health, motivation and habit. Before you started on anything glamorous, I suggested you should check with the
doctor, dentist and opthalmologist. It was to be a long
time before it occurred to anyone that women, especially
if they were married, couldn't afford to pay for beautiful
teeth and eyes.

Irish Beauty was designed as a hard-cover annual with
pages sold to advertisers. It didn't sell. Just as well, for
though it was a good book of its kind, I lost interest in the
subject after it was published. I was beginning to realise
that women's looks were fashioned in the image of man's
fantasy, though I still did not grasp how anyone could ever
do entirely without the beauty and fashion business.
Maybe it was frivolous — and my, what a bunch of Puritans
we were in the Gaj's group for a while! — but I, personally,
needed frivolity and tried to support its importance in the
lives of women with worthy motivations. To deal with the
neurosis of the whole obsession with looks, I got Mary
Kenny to write an article on make-up. She did an ideal job,
explaining how one could become neurotic about facing

the world bare-faced, but that if make-up could be seen as fun, as face-paint which didn't have to be in place every time one's nose went out of doors, then why not? Mary was all for basic skin hygiene, health and fun. It was the last article in the book and I felt that if egos had been battered up to that point, Kenny's article would put it all into perspective.

Beauty, then, was a combination of good fun and good health. But the real split thinking in the book had nothing to do with women's approach to those things. The split was mine. At work I spent hours in the company of the gurus of the beauty and fashion business, while in the group, and in my own reading, I was rejecting all that. In an effort to take the harm out of "straight" beauty and fashion advice I introduced articles such as "Beloved Beauties". It was written by a friend with an interest in poetry and poets, Jean O'Connor, who would never come to a meeting in Gaj's with me, but was *not* responsible for the intro to her article which read: "Woman is always beautiful when she is loved and the beauty of a woman beloved of a great man becomes a legend in Ireland's history; feminine loveliness high-lights with colour and poetry the stories of our heroes." I wrote that, may God and Jean forgive me, because I thought it put the required masculine emphasis on feminine beauty. But the beauties themselves were less insipid. There was Deirdre, "the love-liest woman in the land" who, rather than take to her bed the aged King Conchubor when her lover Naisi was killed, drove a knife into her heart, and Dervorgilla who cast such a spell on Dermot McMurrough that he abducted her from her husband Tiernan O'Rourke of Breffni. There was Dean Swift's *Journal To Stella* which extolled her beauty and womanly virtues on each of her birthdays from thirty to forty-three. I remember thinking that Swift might have found it difficult to praise her beyond that age, had she lived to sag and fall asunder. There were Elizabeth and Maria Gunning, celebrated eighteenth-century beauties, daughters of a poor Roscommon farmer. Their ambitious mother presented them at the Birthnight Ball of 1750 decked out by a friend who was a theatrical costumier. They were so beautiful that crowds in London followed them wherever they walked. Maria became the Countess of Coventry and her sister, Elizabeth married two dukes, the Duke of Hamilton when she was nineteen and, as a forty-year-old widow, the Duke of Argyll.

Beauteous companions of national heroes naturally included Robert Emmet's Sarah Curran, and Parnell's Kitty O'Shea. Then, of course, there was Maude Gonne, enshrined by Yeats as the epitome of Irish beauty. Shaw described her as "outrageously beautiful", and Katherine Tynan in her memoirs said: "When one met her walking in a Dublin street one felt as if a goddess had come to earth." I had met Maude Gonne myself when I was seventeen, and seeing her regal in full-length black velvet was yet appalled at the ravages time had made on her poetic beauty. At seventeen, time seemed to me to be the only enemy of which I was aware and the sight of that great woman did nothing to soothe my horror of old age.

This, then, was the historical sisterhood of Irish beauty. Glamorous to the last, I tottered up the stairs from Gaj's restaurant on high-heeled laced-to-the-knee purple suede boots, behind a mask of make-up. To the younger women in that room I must have looked like an archetypal pre-women's movement dinosaur. Looking at their un-styled hair, clean faces, jeans and comfortable shoes, the uniform of protest in which it was possible to poster, climb and march, I marvelled at their courage in taking on the world dressed like that. I *needed* lipstick. Looking back I would describe my appearance as "hysterical". Even the suburban people in the group didn't look as got up as me. Nell was later to admit that I looked like a dolly-bird which she couldn't understand because she knew I was no teenager. It was a look of the 'fifties, I suppose. Post-war femininity, influenced by Hollywood. My projection of femininity. Me in drag.

In the world outside that room there was a lot going on in the international women's movement. Groups were springing up everywhere. *Shrew* was an amazingly militant publication put out by the London Women's Liberation Workshop, which consisted of several groups. *Shrew* was "6d. for women and 9d. for men until equal pay." In London's Underground I saw the first of those small notices, now commonplace, stuck over advertisements which used the female body or insulted women: "You Earn More As A Real Whore."

1970 brought Germaine Greer, who declared that she was not a feminist, that feminists were grotesque, posturing. She did however, admit that women had been conned; what they wanted was more and better sex, she stated. I couldn't agree more. I still did not understand quite what she meant. Greer's book *The Female Eunuch* was a marvellous text. For me, it made my explorations in the Gaj group especially jell, in regard to what she said about cosmetics and fashion. She was the perfect answer to those who accused us of being a bunch of unattractive, frowsy, ill-kempt women. The crime levelled against us was that we were unfeminine. Here was Greer, tall, fair, blatantly sexy, beautiful and writing: "I'm sick of the masquerade. I'm sick of pretending eternal youth. I'm sick of belying my own intelligence, my own will, my own sex. I'm sick of peering at the world through false eyelashes, so everything I see is mixed with a shadow of bought hairs; I'm sick of weighting my head with a dead mane, unable to move my neck freely, terrified of rain, of wind, of dancing too vigorously in case I sweat into my lacquered curls. I'm sick of the Powder Room. I'm sick of pretending that some fatuous male's self-important pronouncements are the objects of my undivided attention. I'm sick of going to films and plays when someone else wants to and sick of having no opinions of my own about either. I'm sick of being a transvestite. I refuse to be a female impersonator. I am a woman, not a castrate."

I delayed letting all of this sink into my brain, delayed releasing it from my heart until *Irish Beauty* was published in 1971. After the launching, cosmetics never meant the same to me again.

Then came the plague of acne, an acne born of rage and

conflict. It covered my face, stung, burned, bloomed, crusted, faded and bloomed again. Skin doctors gave me the sort of advice I could have got from *Irish Beauty*. Eventually, I found Austin Darragh, a doctor who actually tested my blood and came back with the answer that I was producing too much androgen, the male hormone, which in turn was producing acne. His understanding, for a male chauvinist, was amazing. He would give me medication, he said, but it was up to me whether I had the acne or not. By now I had been living with it for three years. It was a matter, he said, of cooling it, not letting my raised consciousness of the status of women make me angry. "If you are going to be furious all the time then you are letting men bring you out in acne, aren't you?" he asked, delighted with himself. And so, gradually, I learned to deal with the rage and the acne went away.

Over in England, Barbara Castle steered her equal pay bill through Parliament. Six hundred people, including men, attended the first National Women's Liberation Conference at Ruskin College, Oxford. English feminists disrupted the Miss World contest, showering the Albert Hall with flour and leaflets. Five women were arrested. Things were really beginning to happen.

9
MAKING A SHOW

We met on Mondays. On the way to Gaj's one week, Mary Sheerin wearily remarked: "Changing the world is quite a chore for a Monday night." More precisely, we were finding out what was wrong with the world. We were trying to be a structureless, leaderless group, following the main organisational method of groups during those developing years of the women's movement. I say "trying", because structurelessness was something none of us knew anything about. It was hearsay ideology. Our desire to be structureless was in simple reaction to what we did know, the societal structures in which we had grown. Everybody agreed to it, theoretically anyway, because each one of us had a desire to feel free.

Predictably, when women got together to change the world, we didn't want to make the same mistakes as men, or imitate their power systems. We'd all had enough of the rigid structures in our society which left us controlled by others. Structurelessness has remained an intrinsic and accepted part of women's liberation ideology simply because it is a beautiful way of attempting growth, a way based on trust, sharing, nurturing of the individual while working for the good of all. It had a freedom much like being in the house alone with other kids with your stern parent out of the way somewhere. It had a natural feel about it, until one recalled that Nature is the greatest tyrant of all. Compared to conventional meetings I'd attended for voluntary work in Canada, these groups felt as if they were being held in the gentle air of a summer's day.

Structurelessness was ideal for consciousness-raising, providing an atmosphere of space for each one in the same space. It was when we approached tasks that we found structure creeping in, underlying our consciousness, and we fought to keep it out. We simply did not understand what it was we were fighting, the nature of a group. Meanwhile there were no officials. Anyone who was willing got a turn at doing everything. It was awkward and confusing and there were always barneys about who was taking on leadership, being élitist, doing things without proper consultation with the group.

The worst crime was to miss a meeting. There was quite a puritanical attitude towards meetings among the socialists, an intolerance of the middle-class demand for Bank Holiday breaks. Early on, I realised that I agreed with much of the ideology of socialism; the have-nots shouldn't be dependent on charitable hand-outs from the capitalist haves. But the socialists were so earnest, often humourless, like stern governesses silently implying that the rest of us were squandering, decadent. In those early days of the 'seventies the worst thing you could be called was "middle-class". I was painfully aware that because I was Jewish, indulged in clothes and make-up and was easily seduced by comfort, I was recognised by those whose good opinion I longed to earn, the socialists, the morally right, as "middle-class". Ironically, I'd been reared more working-class than most of them, but having been married to a doctor didn't help my image. I thought then I was becoming a socialist, but in recent years when Mavis Arnold of the Women's Political Association phoned me, stuck for a speaker at one of their meetings, and asked: "June, are you a socialist or a capitalist?" I replied "neither, I'm a feminist."

At those meetings we argued over and over again as to what was feminist or merely socialist. Were women being infiltrated by socialist groups? In retrospect, that obsession with whether there were Reds in our midst or whether some of us were hopelessly middle-class is amusing. Of course there was a socialist "infiltration", but sure wasn't there an infiltration of every other political male ideology or lack of it? After all, whether you were right wing, left wing or liberal, it was only trailing after what the boys had decided upon anyway. Nobody, for instance, could have been more Fine Gael than Nuala Fennell, who was to become one of that party's TDs, but wasn't her father a party member before her?

The arguments — and they were exciting, informative — were not merely based on a difference of second-hand political perspective, but part of a developmental process in which most of us needed to find ourselves. Those who were not conscious of what lay ahead for the women's movement in the world, or were not inspired, would go down their own roads in partial commitment. Some would take a middle road, managing to live in a male chauvinist world. Some, like myself, would forever be uncomfortably aware of their position in a society run by men for men. That time left me ever obsessed with the problem of human emancipation, especially my own. Day by day I learned to struggle with the cobweb of societal "norms" which contrives to make everything run smoothly for "them", eating away at the possibility of my personal sense of autonomy. And so, each day, I battle against the little things, those things that grind away the things of which so many women are oblivious, but which none the less contribute to their oppressed status as second class citizens in occupied country.

It was the socialists' impatience with personal indulgence which brought about the agreement to split consciousness-raising off from our weekly planning and business meetings. They were held after the "real" meetings so that you could leave then and not bother taking part. The questions raised varied from "why did you join the women's movement?" — invariably that brought "I wanted to help women less fortunate than myself" from the conservatives — through people like Mary Anderson who declared "because I'm pissed off being buggered in this man's world", to people like me who could not articulate until years later that it was because I wanted to find out what was that weight that pressed upon me. Other topics for consciousness-raising were "how do you think your life would have been different if you'd been born a boy?" and most memorable of all: "what was your reaction when you first saw a penis?" The reactions to that varied from a shrug to high trauma.

When it was my turn to tell about the first time I saw a penis I surprised myself by bursting into tears, bitter and confused. It was a strange experience, the like of which I have since recognised in books on psychotherapy, simply a total recall of feelings around a particular event, years later. The event had been long forgotten, even its memory a surprise to me. Now, here I was sitting opposite Margaret Gaj with her tin box on her ample lap into which she had put our weekly two-shilling pieces and that look in her eye which said: "You all think you invented sex." But there I was, feeling child-sized. No, I was actually child-sized in myself. I was sobbing, confused, breathless with fury. I sobbed the way a toddler does at unexpected insult and Máire Woods took me out of the room in an effort to console me and find out what was the matter. I remember registering that Máire was a doctor, so that I must have gone beyond the pale if she was taking charge. Máire was unshocked by this neurotic outburst, looking sympathetic when I described my first encounter with a penis, but obviously not understanding the sobbing and distress. I couldn't explain to her the feeling that I had fallen back in time, to my three-year-old self. I didn't recognise what had happened until hours later. Now, I told her how some man, perhaps a baby sitter, had thrust his penis through the bars of my cot and I, having been to the Zoo that Sunday afternoon, grabbed it and said: "that's like a snake" and laughed as I wagged the friendly thing up and down. The owner of the penis — and I realise I could probably remember who it was if I really wanted to — smacked my hand hard and said I was a dirty little girl. I was hurt and very surprised. I bawled at the injustice of it. He'd started the game but now I was bad for playing it. It was my first lesson in how men make sex dirty and blame women for it. The incident had disappeared for over thirty years and there in Gaj's that night, I felt the little body of information loosen itself inside me, becoming so alive that even the awareness of my own body changed to the way it was then. I remember feeling I was wearing a diaper and was standing on the soft cot mattress.

In 1971, the Women's Liberation Movement gave birth to a document, *Chains or Change* which was brought forth after much wrangling to preserve structurelessness. It drew up six demands: equal pay, equality before the law, equal education, contraception, justice for deserted wives, unmarried mothers and widows. *Chains or Change* detailed discrimination against women in Ireland. It shocked even some of those who had contributed to its research. Things were even worse for Irishwomen than we had thought, and we still hadn't had the Report on the Commission for the Status of Women. There was much fuss over the demand proposed by Máirín de Burca (who was then so active with the Dublin Housing Action Committee), for one family, one house. Mary Kenny, Nuala Fennell and others were exercised by this Sinn Féin demand, but Máirín swayed a sizeable acceptance of it when she argued that equality would mean little to women who didn't have any kind of decent living accommodation. Woman's place in Ireland was still in the home, so bad housing affected her more than anyone else.

I was divorced by the time I joined the movement, carrying with me a deep-seated horror of the negative possibilities of marriage for a woman. But nothing ever influenced my decisions against remarriage as surely as did the information in *Chains or Change*. Not that remarriage is that common in Ireland, where there is no divorce and Catholics are not permitted to marry divorcées anyway. The common way round that in Ireland is "let's pretend". It's a facade which serves a social, if not legal purpose. And everybody else pretends too that the woman has not merely changed her name by deed poll, so we call them Mr. and Mrs. Same-Name. Deed-poll marriage is remarriage

Irish style, without benefit of divorce in between. All over Dublin you meet deed-poll marriages who could probably, by dint of numbers, influence a move to legalise divorce if only they were prepared to stop pretending and join the Divorce Action Group. Remarriage Irish style leaves a woman's legal rights rather vague, not to mention the status of the children of the union, but sure as long as nobody lets on, it's all right. Remarriage Irish style is not considered the same thing at all as Living in Sin, which brings me back to *Chains or Change.*

The pamphlet contained a brilliant summary by Mary Maher: "Five Good Reasons Why It Is Better To Live In Sin." It has served consistently through the years to remind me to examine why I should ever take a subservient position to any man, in sin or otherwise. Like a bit of knitting, this article has remained cast on the needles of my consciousness. Occasionally I add a line such as "why should I worry about his work ahead of my own, his washing if he doesn't do mine, his food if he won't learn to cook." I'm knitting an invisible garment which looks as if it will not be finished until the day I die. Sometimes I have to unravel a bit of this knitting, but since it is invisible ...

The first reason for living in sin was that you could keep your job. If, in 1970, you were in the Civil Service or semi-State employment, or working for the trade unions or the banks, you'd be expected to resign when you announced your marriage date. You might get re-hired, but on their terms. In some places, it meant you would be on a temporary week-to-week hire basis as the company needed you. It would probably mean far less pay in a lower grade. "If you're in the Civil Service, you and the man you decided not to marry can have two children and you'll still be able to keep your job; you will have a maternity leave of several months." Marriage, on the other hand, meant compulsory retirement until the children were old enough for a woman to find part-time work. Even now, in 1982, the lack of crèches or child-care facilities in Ireland makes it impossible for most women even to contemplate working after they become mothers. "So fifteen years from now you'll find yourself back in the labour force, probably not in a trade union, and therefore unable to fight dismissal, low pay, poor conditions."

The second reason for living in sin was that the Irish tax system at the time discriminated against marriage by making married women pay more tax than single women (a rather hilarious anomaly recently cured by a constitutional case in the courts). Reason number three was that marriage wiped out a woman's commercial identity: opening accounts, taking out insurance, buying on the hire-purchase, borrowing money, all these would require the husband's signature, as a married woman counted only as an infant in Irish law. Even gynaecological operations in some hospitals required the husband's written consent. Meanwhile, a married woman had no right to get any money at all from the selfsame husband: even the children's allowance was paid to him, not her!

All very practical reasons for living in sin. But the fourth and fifth reasons, Mary admitted, were unlikely to be taken seriously by any woman on the brink of marriage, because she would be unwilling to think too deeply about the possibility of the relationship going sour. "A woman who is only living in sin can remember reason number four: you can leave when things have finally become unbearable, merely by walking out the door. A married woman who leaves her husband is presumed to have deserted him and has no right to his home, furniture or income." Which brought us to number five: "If you live in sin you don't submit to the insult that society offers women who marry — the status of property. An adult and equal relationship is something two people forge together. The institution of marriage is something invented to preserve male superiority and a system of female chattels."

How many sinners did this document create?

In spite of Mary Anderson's reading lists, which were circulated for buying and borrowing, we were far from agreed at this stage on what feminist demands should be. And in the midst of that confusion there was dissatisfaction with the élitism which popped up regularly. Some people

charged that people like Mary Kenny, Mary Maher, myself
and other journalists were using the movement as a
personal ego trip. Another dissatisfaction was with the fact
that we were a middle-class bunch, well-off compared to
many women. Hilary Boyle, as I remember, was particularly
concerned on this score. Nuala Fennell, whose thinking
was establishment and organised, was bemused by
structurelessness, seemed ever-conscious of time awasting.
She wanted to achieve something specific, as soon as
possible, on behalf of Irishwomen, preferably with herself
at the helm. A practical person, she was not at all concerned with developing consciousness and turning women
on so much as with obvious jobs to be tackled under her
nose. Some people wanted to expand, to get other people
active, to become a national organisation, but Máirín de
Burca, Mary Maher, Margaret Gaj and Máire Woods felt
that this would be biting off more than we could chew.
Most of us didn't understand anything about structures or
tactics, or how to organise without becoming just another
women's club. I, by that stage, was getting a bid fed up
with structurelessness and its tendency to immobilise. I
wished to heaven that Mary Maher, for instance, wouldn't
insist on being so damn democratic!

Mary Kenny, myself and a few others were impatient to
go public. Mary, because she was such a public person in
those days, could hardly believe that anything actually *was*
until its existence was written and talked, listened and
read. If the media hadn't existed, she'd have invented the
bush telegraph. Headlines crystallised reality for her. For
my part, I have a natural bent which, had I been reared a
Christian, would have landed me in the foreign missions. I
desperately wanted to spread the word. I could talk about
nothing else but women's liberation. I had become an
intrusive fisher of women. An accuser of men. Also, I felt
that the only way to go ahead was to go ahead.

It was during this phase of indecision that attendance
started to fall off a bit, that one clique at least used to
come to meetings determined to manipulate calm, try to
get things running smoothly. The meetings had got to feel

a bit like the Irish sea on a summer's day, fearsome to think about, but lovely when you were in. All hell broke loose the night Mary Kenny turned up saying that she thought it was all set for us to appear on the "Late Late Show" — she thought she could swing the entire show being devoted to women's liberation. The immediate reaction was fury. There she was, ego-tripping again. Who said we wanted to go on television? And if we did, sure as hell Mary Kenny wasn't going to be the self-appointed leader. Who did she think she was? Mary could always handle the mob and explained in that ladylike voice she used for manipulative purposes that Pan Collins, researcher on the "Late Late", had rung her at home, out of the blue, of course, and she had simply chatted to Pan and agreed to have Pan come along to a meeting. Provided we were all willing, naturally. At least an hour was spent discussing the pros and cons of having Pan Collins come to a meeting. How could one trust the "Late Late", especially Gay Byrne, not to use us and abuse us, make a circus out of the whole happening? We could, Kenny assured us, because we would see to it that it was done the way we wished. We'd structure it, choose the speakers, make it an interesting and informative show and not allow ourselves to be baited by Byrne.

I wasn't there the night Pan went along to a meeting of the sisterhood. A few years later when I joined her as a researcher on the "Late Late" team I wondered how she had felt about her meeting with this weird crew of Irish-women. Pan, with her Victorian manners and notions of how to get change without being offensive, must have cringed that night at the uncompromising talk, blue jeans and "unfeminine" approach as to how we would get what we wanted from Gay Byrne. Pan has always been careful of the male ego, and wouldn't ask for a receipt in a pub when entertaining a man for RTE, for fear of slighting his manhood in front of the waiter. She looked at me blankly when I asked what about the female ego? Her ability to turn the other cheek may well be the card that plays her into heaven. Most unacceptable of all militants to Pan was the woman who recognised the male as enemy. She saw no excuse for that. Couldn't women just get on quietly with achieving what they wanted? Yes, she admitted to me, she was a bit disgusted by the group. But she would also have been delighted. The more outrageous was our behaviour in those days when we had newly found voices, the worse the language, the more "unseemly" the appearance, the surer she'd have been that she'd struck oil for the "Late Late" show. Here was a ready-made circus. We could be depended upon to rant and rave, forget the camera, entertain the viewers, bring in showers of protesting letters, keep Gay Byrne happy. She'd have disliked the sinners, loved our sins. For the purposes of television. Pan is a true professional. The result of her visit was that Gay Byrne offered to devote an entire show to women's liberation on 6 March 1971.

He wasn't going to have it all his own way, though. It was finally agreed, through Mary Kenny, that the women's movement would organise the programme and choose speakers. He wasn't taking much of a risk since Mary Kenny was the media success of the day and was orchestrating the whole thing with a very capable journalist backing her up. We printed leaflets announcing the show (a total breach of "Late Late" policy) and the points which would be discussed in it. Unequal pay, the civil service marriage ban, tax, children's allowances, jury service — the lot.

We were going to use that greatest user of people, the "Late Late Show", to get our own show off the ground. In a way, the offer of the show had forced us to become a mass movement, and we would be ruthless in addressing ourselves to the women of Ireland, the hell with Gay Byrne or RTE. For a structureless, leaderless group we certainly did a good job of structuring that Saturday night. Nothing was left to chance, we teased out every thread. We planned to present ourselves at our most acceptable, informed, rational, even moderate. Mary Kenny, for all her orchestrating behind the scenes, was ordered to keep a low profile, as were other personalities who were known to TV

160

viewers. At one point it was a question of whether we would even be permitted to take a place in the audience. A bunch of us met Gay Byrne and company for breakfast at the Montrose Hotel the week before the show to make final arrangements. There was even a hassle over that. Breakfast? Pan explained that this was 1971 and people everywhere were meeting for breakfast to lengthen the day.

We didn't have a legal brain in the group and had been trying to get Senator Mary Robinson to join us for some time. Now, however, she agreed to appear on the TV panel to point out the legal inequities and how they betrayed the Constitution of Ireland. Mary Cullen, the historian who years later founded the Women's Study Group in Maynooth College under the auspices of the Irish Foundation for Human Development, was invited to make the case for working mothers. Gay Byrne introduced her as the wife of a psychiatrist. Lelia Doolin, one of Ireland's very few TV producers, who had co-authored the book *Sit Down and be Counted* presented our views on the education or miseducation of girls, and on social conditioning, with particular reference to the media. Máirín Johnston took her place on the panel to talk about discrimination at work and jobs barred to women, and urged all women to join trade unions. Máirín had been doing that in "real life" since she was a teen-ager working in Dublin sweatshop factories, and was forever losing jobs because she tried to organise the other girls into unions. Nell McCafferty made the case for women without men — although she didn't put it like that — when she spoke for deserted wives, unmarried mothers and widows. At the time, the deserted wives' allowance was £4 a week given on the basis of Home Assistance, a Poor Law provision, and there was nothing at all for the unmarried mother.

The rest of us who had contributed to writing *Chains or Change* were armed with facts in the audience. Mary Earls and myself had spent that afternoon photostatting the pamphlet. My special brief that night was unmarried mothers. I didn't know even one unmarried mother in

Dublin at the time, proof of how attitudes drove them underground. But I identified with being a single parent, an unmarried mother. Wasn't I a mother of three and unmarried? Nobody else agreed with this view of my status. In any case, I knew of the terrible fears that existed around pre-marital sex among Irishwomen in Dublin. I knew about the awful baby homes where they made mothers give their babies up for adoption. How could you possibly keep it anyway? I knew of the flight of the wild geese to give birth in England or to have abortions. Wasn't I entitled to be called a wild goose myself? I identified so much with unmarried mothers in those days that eventually when "Cherish" was organised for the single parent by Maura O'Dea and I applied for membership, I was deeply hurt to be rejected on the grounds of having been married before I became a mother.

The same discussion on Irish television now would be a switch-off. It's all been said, by so many different people. But then it was new. The reasonable moderate tone of the show was maintained, much like a documentary, while each panellist had her say, some speaking for a surprisingly long time. The strategy came unstuck when the audience was invited to join in. By then, we were all itching in our seats anyway. Even more surprising than the audience's rapt attention while the panel rabbitted on was the way in which Gay Byrne handled the show. He was dispassionate, objective, the perfect impartial chairman. Once or twice, he even stepped out of his rôle onto our side. For a long time after that I judged him as one of those men who enjoy the breasts of both worlds — career and home — providing they packaged themselves like models and were never, ever boring. By all means be a nuclear physicist, but have you the legs to go with it? He's come a long way ... and he played fair that night. He examined, picked apart, every page of *Chains or Change,* giving members of the audience the chance to ask questions, to make a point. Strangely, it was Nuala Fennell who struck the first crusty note. In those days Nuala often sounded cross and looked angry. She was obsessed with the helpless dependency of the Irish wife, particularly in relation to finance and desertion. Hers was an externalised feminism. She never looked at the institution of marriage, questioned whether people should or should not get married.

Nuala asked Mary Robinson how article 41 of the Constitution could be reconciled with the fact that there was no machinery here to safeguard the provision of an adequate and regular house-keeping allowance to a wife? She pointed out the significance of 11% of personal income in Ireland being spent on alcohol. This was the highest amount spent in Europe, yet most European countries had machinery to make sure that a wife got a fair share of her husband's pay. She outlined the position in other countries, asking how we could get this legislation here.

At this point a woman in the audience said that often an unemployed man drank all the money he got on the dole, and without having to change the Constitution it ought to be possible to have a local committee to whom the wife could complain, and the money could then be given directly to her. "Do you really think, seriously, that a patriarchal society is going to do this? Do you really think that the men in Dáil Éireann, the men who make the legislative situation in this country, care at all?" asked Mary Kenny, smiling sarcastically at the notion. "I think that they would drag their heels, they would resist changes in any of these areas up to the hilt, because I don't think that they give a damn."

Mary Robinson went on to point out that the answer to that was the fact that so many Irish citizens and voters were women. The woman in the audience came in again, asking if there was an Attorney General's Office in Ireland where one could go, as in the States, to say you were being discriminated against because you were a woman? Was there a Department of Justice? she asked.

"There *is* a Department of Justice ..." Senator Robinson began, but laughter from the audience made it impossible for her to continue. Then Gay gave the floor to a "gentleman at the back". He said that if Mary Kenny wanted support for women's liberation, she would have to point out to men why it would suit them because that was the best way to get support. "I would ask any of the males who think that women's liberation is none of their business, think of it, if they have a wife at home, or daughters at home, and if tomorrow they were to die, these women would not be allowed to earn to their full potential and they have the potential."

I'd been seething for ages. It seemed to me that everyone thought some other woman was oppressed, not herself. That other men were doing the oppressing, not himself. When my turn came to speak, I said that in Ireland you didn't have to be black to be discriminated against, you just had to be a woman. I attacked the complacency of women, the fact that when I talked about equality or liberation, the deafest people were well-heeled women who believed in the happily-ever-after marriage fairy tale. They didn't believe they could ever be deserted or that their daughters might be unmarried mothers.

Anger made my words crowd each other. A man had yelled "Oh, come off it" when I'd claimed that women in Ireland were the ones most discriminated against. Now Gay asked him to expand on that. Said Mr. X: "I don't believe women are discriminated against. I think the Irishman is always a gentleman and always will be." There was a howl from the audience and Gay Byrne asked: "Have you another blinding flash of brilliance?"

Then there followed the inevitable argument about Ireland being a subject nation, a victim of colonialism, and how could women be free until Ireland was set free? Gay brought us back to the point by referring to the day's editorial in *The Limerick Leader*, reading aloud: "The four thousand or so men of Leichtenstein decided this week that their tiny alpine principality should remain the only European country where women may not vote. There is a strong temptation to smile, but one need not look to an obscure corner of the Continent for examples of male madness. Consider for example, the way in which Mrs. Frances Quillinan, of Limerick, is being treated by officialdom. For 11 years this talented mother of four, of Mill Road, Corbally, has been a member of the Corporation's architectural staff. Last May she became senior architect in a temporary capacity. Recently, she applied for the permanent post that was advertised but was not even granted an interview. Why? Because she married and became thereby automatically ineligible for the position."

Frances Quillinan was in the audience and confirmed that she was not even allowed to contest the job because she was a married woman, under Section 16 of the Local Government Act of 1955. Her credentials would certainly qualify her for the job had she been a man or a single or widowed woman. And they were having trouble filling the post. Perhaps, if they absolutely couldn't find a suitable man, then Frances Quillinan would be considered for the left-over job.

The temperature continued to rise. In spite of all the care taken with planning the show, the panel was enlarged in a most unexpected way during the commercial break. Garret FitzGerald, Fine Gael TD, roused by Mary Kenny's remarks about legislators, had dashed from his fireside and presented himself at RTE for an appearance on the show. A researcher ushered him into the studio and those of us who realised what had happened were sitting in the audience, pretty furious. In the first place, it was obvious then that such a take-over could only happen on a woman's programme, and also that we were to be used in a band-wagon bid for country-wide publicity for the Fine Gael Party. Nobody was ever allowed to appoint themselves to a "Late Late" panel before then, and certainly never during my years on the "Late Late". However, the dramatic potential of such an intervention was too good to be passed up. Had I been working for the show there that night, I'd have been delighted to see him.

Gay introduced him as "one of your hated legislators". Garret FitzGerald said that fury had got him from his fireside to confront Mary's reference to TDs. The assumption that legislators would only work for change if they personally would benefit offended Garret. "Okay, you can accuse your TDs of lots of things, the fact that a lot of these reforms haven't been carried out suggests laziness, and lack of interest, but don't assume that it is a vested interest. People aren't like that, the legislators aren't like that. If these reforms haven't come about it's because the system responds to pressure, all kinds of pressure, and there haven't been pressures in this area. There hasn't been pressure for civil rights from women."

A free-for-all screaming match followed between Garret FitzGerald and various women in the audience. Gay suggested that we "behave like gentlemen, for God's sake." I remember screaming: "Ah, so now it's a man's show. The bosses take over." Someone pulled my skirt and when I sat down the seat was up and I landed with a bump on the floor. Garret continued: "When you say that legislators aren't doing anything, I spent a fair bit of time last Tuesday, I'm not supposed to say this, I'll be shot for saying it, with John Kelly, in drafting a bill covering these very things you are talking about."

"Which ones, which ones?" I called.

"The maintenance of deserted wives."

Mary Kenny broke in: "Garret, there is one point to make. You are not the government, as you are well aware."

"Wait, let me finish. One suggestion was that we should treble the limit. And we agreed that this one is quite inadequate, that what should be done in a case like this is that if a wife is deserted and there are no children, the husband should have to pay up to half of his income, and for children, up to two-thirds."

Nell interrupted: "As it stands at the moment, if the wife goes out to work, the measly benefits she gets are withdrawn immediately."

"All these reforms *will* be carried out. That's only one thing that we've dealt with," said this TD, not then in a position to carry out any reforms at all. He then pointed out that the opposition in parliament could not introduce any bill that involved a charge on the exchequer. Mary Maher was not satisfied with that excuse: "They can vote against repressive legislation. Why isn't Fine Gael voting against the Forcible Entry Bill? It's the working women who want houses; vote against repressive legislation!"

"This is not fair," I protested.

Gay: "What is not fair?"

Me: "This is not a political platform."

Nell rolled up her sleeves as if she was going to fight, and launched into a speech as fluent as any of Dr. FitzGerald's: "Garret said he doesn't want to go back, he wants to enter into this year, and he says he has made a speech and I would like to say that the present Bill coming through in 1971, the response to social pressure for houses in this country, is that the government is going to introduce a bill whereby any man who in desperation squats in a house will be jailed, his wife will be jailed; Garret FitzGerald knows, everybody knows that the Government will pass that bill because they are in the majority; speeches are not enough. If Garret FitzGerald is so responsive to social pressures, I look forward to Garret FitzGerald joining the women of the country on the day that bill becomes law and I look forward to seeing him break the law. I want to see him in that first house where that first woman is going to be put into jail, in response to the social pressure put on that woman. Let's have his actions where his mouth is."

Garret assured her: "I'm with you a hundred per cent, Nell!"

"Then vote against the bill."

Garret began explaining the party difficulty about voting against the bill, but promised to oppose every clause in the Bill.

Gay asked Máire Woods to get us back to Women's Liberation, and Máire insisted that we should not think for a moment that we could free women, or indeed men, by saying the words "women's liberation". That implied that men were the exploiters, said Máire. "It's not men who are the exploiters, it's the capitalist system." She was interrupted by a woman who said that women in Ireland had a servile attitude. She had personally liberated herself, she said, by doing a six week's course in a modelling, poise and charm school. At this, there were screams from the audience. Another woman stated that she belonged to a recently formed group called the Women's Progressive Association, which aimed to encourage women to take a more active rôle in public life, particularly in politics. Until women got out and did this, she said, there was no way of speeding up the elimination of the discriminatory situation against women. She asked every woman to join a political party.

A strong voice came in from the back of the studio: "All these women want is to be treated as responsible human beings. To be able to develop in whatever way we want. To be able to work, to have the right to work, whether we're married or single, black or white, or whatever our creed may be. That I think, is the most important thing, and to change the climate of opinion against us. We in our association have protested against unequal pay, and we have had letters from semi-state bodies saying that it is the custom and practice in this country. I feel the women in the homes are largely responsible for the position we are in today, because children are conditioned from the moment they are born by discrimination in the home, and human rights begin in the home and I feel that women themselves must change their thinking."

The Women's Progressive Association had been formed by Councillor Margaret Waugh of Dun Laoghaire who, legend has it, travelled around the borough from door to door on her bicycle recruiting women who she thought might take an interest in public life. The association's name was later changed to the Women's Political Association.

The audience was well laced with socialists, Marxists and Nationalists who argued back and forth about it all being the fault of capitalism or British imperialism. One woman pointed out that the British TUC first put in a claim for equal pay as far back as 1886 and challenged Garret FitzGerald over his claim that there had been no pressure for civil rights from Irishwomen. Garret came in again to insist that there hadn't been the type of concerted pressure from women that came from the farmers, industry and other sectors. Until we put on that kind of pressure we wouldn't get results. The fat was in the fire again, with women yelling and attacking Garret for turning the show into a party political broadcast.

As the angry voices died down, the manipulative voice of the oppressed came from a woman in the audience: "Gay, there has been an awful lot of grousing, I know that in this country there are an awful lot of under-privileged women, but surely amongst us to-night there must be a few women who are happily married and have babies, who were elevated when they had those babies, liberated, call it what you want ..." Before the storm rose again Gay Byrne said we'd have to pack it in, mentioning that a bouquet of flowers had come for Mary Kenny, and that as she was one of the main organisers of the show he would ask her to wrap it up. She took up the political point once again: "I actually think that Fine Gael's policy on women is the best of the three parties, but I do think that most people seem to act in their own interests. I agree with you that nobody has put pressure on the legislators to make these changes in inequities for women and that depends entirely on women in this country getting together and doing so, but that's where liberation comes in because they won't get together and do so until the inequities have been removed, until the social condition of women has changed and until the whole system has changed. They will stay home passively, they're safe, they're married, they don't care about other people. That's where liberation comes in and that's where we're going to start. We're going to start living and making it hard for you."

* * *

The socialists weren't satisfied that the discussion on the Forcible Entry Bill had got sufficient airing, the others were dissatisfied that the discussion had veered away from women for so much of the time. Most of the Gaj's group felt that Garret FitzGerald had pulled a fast one. Remarks about the source of Mary Kenny's flowers caused her to refuse to reveal who had sent them. She never did tell.

Whether the show got away from us or not, it served its purpose. Now, the women of Ireland had a fair clue as to what we were about.

The show had been chaotic in spite of all the orchestration. Almost everything we had planned to avoid had happened. Mary Kenny had got shrill, the rest of us hadn't exactly kept our cool, the Marxists had taken up valuable time, a man had stolen the limelight.

It had, after all, been a typical "Late Late" of that spontaneous, compulsive-viewing quality that made that show the most popular and the longest-running in the country. OK, so it had been a circus. We'd jumped through the hoops of our own accord, but we had been given ample opportunity to present *Chains or Change* before the free-for-all. Having educated people as to what we were about, we might then have cancelled ourselves out with the boredom of prolonged discussion. Some of the plain people of Ireland might have been shocked by what was afterwards described again and again as our "unfeminine carry-on", but at least they hadn't switched off. The "Late Late" had delivered Women's Liberation to the women of Ireland.

Now the pamphlet was thoroughly reviewed in the national newspapers. We became the female gurus of the 'seventies with all the attendant pros and cons of such a rôle. Like it or not, and some did and some did not, we *were* women's liberation. We set about organising our first mass meeting, the now famous Mansion House event which packed the Round Room of the Lord Mayor of Dublin's residence with over 1,000 people, mostly women. When Mary Sheerin booked the Round Room, she told me it looked *huge* and that Wednesday night, 14 April 1971, it looked so small and inadequate.

In the meantime, two things were happening: There was heated public discussion of Mary Robinson's contraceptive bill, introduced for the first time in the Senate, and the fight against the pending Forcible Entry Bill was gathering speed. I had become obsessed with the latter, and had written about it in my weekly column in the *Sunday Independent*. The harshness of this Bill directed against the homeless, its mindless cruelty, shocked me. I was happy to write and demonstrate and march against this legislation to the point where I was finding it difficult to give equal energy to the Irish Women's Liberation Movement.

On the last Sunday in March I straggled along to Mass in the Pro-Cathedral for the purpose of walking out in high dudgeon. The protest was in response to a letter, condemning contraception from the then Archbishop of Dublin, Dr. McQuaid, and the priests were reading it to the congregations that Sunday. As a teen-age reporter I had met the Archbishop, and he had offered me his ring to kiss. Being officially Jewish, I declined, and the Archbishop had put his hand on my head and said: "Bless you, my child," and something in Latin. Then, later, he had personally seen to it that I had refreshments.

The Saturday night before the protest, I had a nightmare in which the Archbishop was speaking from the pulpit and suddenly spied me kneeling behind a pillar. He just shook his head sadly. I lay in bed that Sunday morning vaguely wary of the possibility of being found out and asked publicly, who cared whether I walked out of church or not? In fact, would I be so kind as to get out? Not that I was the only one taking part in that protest who had rarely been inside a church. Some women went to Mass several times that day so that they could walk out, but once was all I could manage. I've always had an awe of sacred places, no matter which religion they belonged to. It's the childhood thing about God being in them. As I marched up the aisle towards the door I felt Eyes on my back! That evening there was a picket on the Archbishop's residence.

Even after the reaction to the "Late Late Show", we weren't prepared for the crowds who came to the Mansion House and it was decided, at the last minute, that a bunch of us should stand behind tables at the door and take women's names and postal districts as they came in. One person from each postal district was asked to organise a meeting to choose representatives to attend the first delegate meeting of Irish Women's Liberation to be held in

Gaj's restaurant a few weeks later.

The meeting was chaired by Nell McCafferty with Máire Woods, Máirín Johnston, Mary Maher, Hilary Orpen of RTE and Ivan Kelly, a solicitor, on the platform. The demands of the movement were outlined and discussed. Then Nell invited the audience to speak from the floor microphone provided. They queued up. At one stage I counted a line of fifty-two people. It was a moving experience. We had known those women were out there, but not so many, so willing to share their life's experiences and their views with us. It was spontaneous sisterhood, the Round Room a power-house of female energy. The sight of them brought me up in goose bumps, the sound of them the ultimate confirmation if we needed it that we Irishwomen needed liberation. It was the first time I'd been to a mass meeting run feminist style, everybody being given time to speak, and if someone was interrupted or cut short, a voice would come from the audience — a different one each time and not one of ours — "let her speak, she's not finished yet." The audience that night seemed to have an instinct for sisterhood. People poured their hearts out and you had the feeling that there would be no gossip about them the next day. They spoke of being widows, or deserted wives wrestling with the law, of starvation, work experiences, contraception and what the lack of it had done or was doing to their marriages. They spoke off the cuff and were articulate and mostly to the point, like friends over a cup of coffee. Among other things, it was to be remembered as the night the first Irish unmarried mother declared herself publicly. I hadn't ever *seen* one before and stretched my neck to get a better look at Helen Heaveny when she stepped up to the mike and said: "I'm an unmarried mother ..." She had to pause while deafening applause encouraged her to go on. She spoke simply, practically, about having her child and rearing it on her own.

Once again, the socialist issue caused disruption when the question of participation in the May Day March was brought up. It was decided that Women's Liberation would march under our own banner. (In the event, three hundred people marched behind the banner, forming about one third of all the marchers). Meanwhile, by the end of the Mansion House meeting most of the group were aware that we had a mammoth job on our hands. De Burca, Maher, Gaj and company had been right. What did we know of structures, tactics, mass organisation?

"Christ," said Nell, before the meeting had even started, "what are we going to do with all these lovely women? They'll expect us to know what to do ..." She covered her face with her hands. They did, indeed, expect us to know what to do. And yet, at the same time, from the beginning, they resented anything that sounded like an "order from headquarters." They wanted leadership, yet they resented being led. Now began the wrangle over structurelessness, in earnest.

Over thirty women, each one representing an area of Dublin, came to that first delegate meeting in Gaj's. Working class districts and fashionable suburbs were represented. Most of them had never met each other before, but from the first meeting, there was this "us" and "them" thing. On the first meeting, "they" insisted on keeping left-wing politics out of women's liberation. They argued over our appearance at the May Day March, but agreed that those who wished could march behind our banner. Some declared flatly that they would have nothing to do with opposing the Forcible Entry Bill, not because they agreed with it, but because it was not, strictly speaking, of specific interest to women. We were being sucked into the service of existing political and pressure groups. However, we certainly all agreed on contraception being a basic issue of women's liberation, most claiming it as the central issue.

Out of that first meeting of delegates came the decision to do something "worthwhile" about it. The use of the Pill was spreading, prescribed by doctors as a cycle regulator, not a contraceptive, and taken doggedly by many women in spite of any unpleasant side-effects or rumoured dangers. An observant visitor to Ireland, perhaps from outer space, could easily have wondered at the medical profile of Irish-women and their dicey reproductive potential. Mechanical contraceptives were used by those who could get them, either through foreign travel or illegally through family planning clinics, wherever there might be such a place.

It's hard to know who had the idea of a contraceptive train full of women who would go to Belfast and buy contraceptives, declaring them at the Irish customs when we came back. Nell McCafferty recalls that during 1970 there was a People's Democracy March from Belfast to Dublin, and at the border the Newry Customs caught "a wee quiff of a boy called Cyril Toman." He held up two things saying: "This is Edna O'Brien's *Country Girl* which has been banned, and this is a Durex and it's not allowed in the South." She had laughed, what with the absurdity of the condom, of which she knew little, and out of shock, thinking "Jesus, what has this to do with Civil Rights?"

By May the following year, she knew right well what contraception had to do with civil rights. The point was that the Contraceptive Law affected those who most needed contraceptives, the poor and women who could not take or get the pill. Anyone who could take the train to Belfast could have all the contraceptives they wanted. The Customs people never bothered about them when they came back to Ireland. The idea of Women's Liberation was to show up the hypocrisy. We would challenge the Customs men which meant they would have to charge us with breaking the law or let us pass, proving the law obsolete.

There was a lot of discussion about the shocking nature of our venture, its likelihood of alienating the very women whom we wished to reach. Should single women go on the train? It was left up to ourselves.

On World Communications Day, 22 May, at 8 o'clock, forty-seven of us turned up to take the train to Belfast from Connolly Station. Our day was to become an international media story, lauded far more elsewhere than it was at home. As well as the national newspaper reporters there were at least four TV cameramen. I was covering the story for the *Sunday Independent* which gave the tale, with pictures, front page headlines and an inside double-page spread. The *Irish Press* had disclaimed interest in sending a photographer; "more important" things were happening in Belfast that day. A man had been shot.

We took over two carriages, and the rest of the train filled with Southern housewives on their way to bargains in Belfast. Mary Maher was in hospital having her baby, Máirín de Burca stayed in Dublin to organise our homecoming, Margaret Gaj was nursing a sick husband and Nuala Fennell felt the whole exercise was counterproductive. Mary Anderson and Nell McCafferty had instruction sheets waiting for us. Literature on contraceptives was waiting for us in Belfast so that we could bring it back with us for confiscation. The sheet informed us that we could get Durex, The Pill, Intrauterine devices (also known as the loop and the coil), and the Dutch Cap (also known as the diaphragm). Unless we had prescriptions, we were told, we must buy spermicidal jelly or Durex (obviously not for your personal use). Spermicidal jelly, we were told, had been consistently confiscated by the customs. We were advised that free legal aid was on tap for everyone. The following choices of action were open to us when confronting the Customs men upon return to Dublin:

1. Declare nothing and risk being searched.
2. Declare contraceptives and refuse to be searched.
3. Declare contraceptives and refuse to hand over.
4. Declare contraceptives and hand over with protest of infringement of your constitutional rights.
5. Declare contraceptives and throw over barrier to sisters waiting beyond. Many people who couldn't come today will be demonstrating at Amiens Street in solidarity with our action.
6. Declare contraceptives and sit down in anticipation of customs action.
7. Declare internal contraceptive. Allow search from Female Officer only and shout "April Fool" before entry.

In the event of being searched between Belfast and Dublin,

we were advised that any of the above actions could mean being detained while the train passed on. In the event of action on points 2, 3 and 5, we could be liable to prosecution and appearance in court.

Another sheet laid out our Constitutional Rights as follows:

> Article 44; subsection 2, para. 1:
> Freedom of conscience and the free profession and practice of religion are, subject to public order and morality, guaranteed to every citizen.

> Article 42; Subsection 1:
> The State acknowledges that the primary and natural educator of the child is the family and guarantees to respect the inalienable right and duty of parents to provide, according to their means, for the religious and moral, intellectual, physical and social education of their children.

> Article 41: Subsection 1:
> The State recognises the family as the natural primary and fundamental unit group of society and as a moral institution possessing inalienable and imprescriptible rights, antecedent and superior to all positive law. The State therefore, guarantees to protect the family as its constitution and authority, as the necessary basis of social order and as indispensable to the welfare of the Nation and the State.

> Article 41: ss 2, par 2.
> The State shall, therefore, endeavour to ensure that mothers shall not be obliged by economic necessity to engage in labour to the neglect of their duties in the home. (This last was followed by an explanation containing an interesting mistake: "This means that if you have more children than you can afford you will be forced to work for a living.")

Article 40, Subsection 6:
The State guarantees liberty for the exercise of the
following rights, subject to public order and morality:
The right of the citizens to express freely their con-
victions and opinions ... The right of the citizens to
assemble peacably and without arms ... The right of
the citizens to form associations and unions ...

The last line promised that each one of us would be
supplied with a pill: "Declare it to the Customs officer and
swallow it."

Those off the train first went, naturally, to the chemist
shop opposite the Europa Hotel near the station. The rest
of us tried to pack noisily in after them. All the relevant
stuff was on display, creating embarrassed titters for some
who had never seen contraceptives. A couple of middle-
aged women standing close to me were acting the way I
felt the first time I went into a sex shop in Soho, trying to
appear impassive, mortified, and undecided whether to
laugh or run. Some had no trouble laughing, it was like the
dirty giggles of naughty children. "Pretty disgusting when
you think about it," said one young woman studying the
instructions on spermicidal cream. She had the pale, clear
looks of West of Ireland ancestry, her sheet of silken black
hair in the way of her reading. It was going to take more
than a visit to a Northern Irish chemist shop to raise *her*
consciousness on the contraceptive issue. She'd be the sort
who'd be surprised that "accidents" cause people.

Whether it was that some women hadn't got leaflets,
hadn't read them or hadn't absorbed the information was
hard to say, but there now followed an amazing display of
ignorance of the facts of life. For reasons I have never
cared to examine, then or later, they cast me as the
authority on such matters and I was pressed with questions
such as "what does gossamer mean?", "what do you do
with this jelly stuff?" and from one woman: "Would I take
the same size Dutch cap as you, d'you think?" A foreign
pressman asked if I were a doctor as a cameraman pushed
his way through to the counter. I had been impressed by

the "newness" of some of these young women of the 'seventies. Now I saw them as their mothers' daughters, women who knew little about their own bodies, who had never been free to feel responsible for their own fertility and felt awkward about it. They handled the condoms as if they were packages of sins, hooted at sight of a diaphragm. Such shopping was foreign to them and a hint of hysteria made them vulgar. At last it was over, some women going to the Family Planning Clinic to find it closed.

I've never seen Belfast before or since as it was that day, alight with spring. As Nell and I walked along there seemed to be tulips, daffodils and crocuses around all the public buildings. "It's the sort of day when something lovely should happen," I remarked, vaguely downed by the scene in the chemist shop.

"Ah well," said Nell, stopping to buy a bunch of pink tulips from a flower seller, "here are six lovely things," and presented me with the tulips. They became an awkward burden as the day wore on but I think then I was a little in love with Nell and the flowers were still with me that night, limp lovelies on the desk beside me, as I wrote my story in Independent House. I put them in water in the wee hours of Sunday morning and they hung exhaustedly over the edge of the vase for days before I threw them out in the field beyond the garden. I never thought of putting them in with the garbage.

Around lunchtime we trailed into a Chinese restaurant, backing off again when we saw a few young women playing with condoms at the table as the waiter took their order. We roamed about the shops, me buying a few things for the children, but when Nell mentioned that she wished she could find clothes to fit her and needed a coat, I got set on finding Nell a coat. As I hauled her round the shops she had the air of a child on a day's outing with her mother, but she couldn't see herself wearing anything I asked her to try on. Finally, her jaw set, she said: "there's no way I'm going to make myself look the way you want me to look," and we gave up on the coat.

For the few hours before the train we kept bumping

into groups from the Contraceptive Train, laden down with bargains. If all was normal on the rest of the train returning home, with 90% of passengers being housewives and working girls smuggling back cheap clothes for themselves and their families, it was tense and hectic in my carriage. One of our members was having morning sickness in the late afternoon for a start. And Mary Kenny had caused such disturbance in another part of the train that one of the organisers came and asked would I please take her in "my" carriage and mind her and not let her get up to anything. It wasn't easy. She was beside herself with excitement and was greatly offending an ordinary passenger sitting opposite with a child. Her chat was unsuitable in front of the child, even though Mary always said the most outrageous things in polite English. I can't remember if the woman left the carriage or not. Certainly, she wrote to the papers the following week saying how disgraceful we had been. It was when Mary started to blow up condoms that I restrained her. She could blow them to a huge balloon size and collapse with laughter as she let go of the end and the thing went shooting around the carriage.

"Mary, come on, what would your mother say?" I pleaded and off she'd go again, blowing the condom up and holding it well out of my reach. Instinctively, I knew worry would calm her down and got her engrossed in the possibility of our venture falling flat on its face. Suppose our pals had already been arrested in Dublin that afternoon for disturbing the peace? Suppose Tim Pat Coogan got really mad this time and sacked her? She went pensive then, asking had I seen the landrovers parked outside the station with soldiers and rifles at the ready? "Poor Northern Ireland," said Mary. She was settled in her seat now, thinking, and I took a walk to the loo. Some of the Saturday shoppers glared at me, others pointedly ignored me, while others were too busy putting on layers of newly-bought clothing or concealing things on their person to notice one way or another. One woman called: "you've great courage, rightly or wrongly you've that itself ..." The women had a right to be mad at us. After all, the customs usually didn't bother housewives and now we were baiting them to search everyone. It was tough luck for them landing on the Contraceptive Train.

There was some talk that the train might be boarded by gardaí at Dundalk, but as we swept through the station we settled down to another fifty miles of freedom. It was about now that Mary amazed me with the remark as she hung out of the window for air: "Our mothers will kill us!" And behind all the bravado, it was a common sentiment. I didn't care, but I realised now that these women would have to face shocked neighbours and friends and bear the brunt of the speeches from the pulpits next day and for weeks afterwards. And speeches there were. Indeed, even as we travelled home, speaking at Knock Shrine, Co. Mayo, the Bishop of Clonfert, the Most Rev. Dr. Ryan, said that never before and certainly not since penal times was the Catholic heritage of Ireland subjected to so many insidious onslaughts on the pretext of conscience, civil rights and women's liberation. We were attacking the principles of the Church's teaching, he said. "The chief targets of attack are the Church's teaching on contraception and divorce and the Church's rôle in the education of youth." He prayed that the Virgin Mary, appointed patroness of telecommunications, would guide the media in Ireland, making us instruments for good and not for evil.

Now we were coming into Dublin, hanging out of the windows and longing for a sign of what was happening at that end. And then, yes, it *was* singing we heard in the distance and a huge number of voices: "We Shall Overcome" brought tears to the eye. I gave up the fear of spending even five minutes in a cell. We'd been scared, but now we'd see it through. The station was a teeming mass of people with banners, cheering. We unfurled our banner, with the Sutton group carrying it, and Colette O'Neill marching in front of it, mother of four, singing at the top of her lungs. The order came: "Loose your contraceptives!" and we slid our packets beyond the feet of the customs men along the platform towards our supporters. The men dropped their eyes, silent and fussed, as a group of us who had decided to declare and not surrender waved our purchases at the customs men, who ignored us and passed us through.

The papers said next day that other women said we should be shot or locked up, but we weren't even arrested. The Government had decided not to enforce the Criminal Law Amendment Act. It took thirty minutes before we knew for sure that the customs men were going to let us pass — they were preoccupied with shoppers. All the time we chanted: "Enforce the Constitution now" and "The law is obsolete." Now we were through the customs with our condoms and other Irish unmentionables. On this occasion, lip service to the law had been paid on a grand scale. Now we marched to Store Street station near by, the crowds after us. We could see the gardaí through their office windows. They didn't even glance out. They pretended we weren't there.

Among the crowds that came to greet us were Rosita Sweetman and her husband. He had just returned from Tanzania that morning, so instead of taking the Contraceptive Train to Belfast, they had spent a happy day in bed. They were with us in spirit.

As we marched along, Myles McWeeney of the "Late Late Show" grabbed Colette O'Neill, who appeared with Mary Kenny on the show that night. Once again there was a chance to tell the nation that those sections of the Constitution guaranteeing the rights of the family and the individual were the basis of the revolt against the law which made the importation of contraceptives an offence, and Dáil Éireann was charged with being "manipulated by forces outside the electorate." The women accused the state of criminal responsibility in leaving thousands of Irishwomen with no choice other than to use the contraceptive pill legally available to them, imported as a "cycle regulator" simply because this was a technical evasion of the law, despite the fact that such ovulants are, in many cases, medically unsuitable and damaging to those women who might otherwise, in all conscience, choose other methods. On World Communications Day, we had certainly succeeded in communicating ... the question was, what would we do for an encore?

It was only when one had time to consider that I realised what an impressive job Máirín de Burca had done in rounding up that overwhelming crowd at Connolly Station. At the time, it looked as if the revolution had come at last.

10
REVOLUTIONARY

"They think you are getting us involved in politics and revolution, Máirín," I said to Máirín de Burca, the Sinn Féin activist, one night.

"They'd be right," said Máirín, "we *are* involved in politics. We're trying to change the things that affect people's lives, that's as political and revolutionary as you can get. What else do you think we're at?"

I had only made the remark for the sake of something to say to Máirín, with whom I'd found myself alone over a cup of tea in Gaj's. I mean, what could you talk to Máirín about? I felt she disapproved of consciousness-raising groups as impractical and a waste of time. And though she was always friendly towards me, I thought that she found me a bit middle-class and high-falutin' in my interests. I couldn't chat with her, being so much in awe of her, the way I could with Mary Kenny, Nuala Fennell and most of the others. She made me feel frivolous. She wasn't really into chat, come to think of it. And so I'd trotted out what people were saying about us.

Maybe I expected her to say "nonsense", but I was certainly unprepared for the effect her answer had. A light seemed to go on for me. Quite suddenly, in the space of time it took to finish the tea I realised that all the "whys" of my life had political answers. No wonder I couldn't find any answer to those "whys". I hadn't known where to look. The more I thought over what Máirín had said — us, revolutionaries — the more I realised that I had always been interested in politics. I had simply never given myself permission to call it that because I thought politics a man's preserve.

There I'd been, a fairly typical woman, pretending politics was nonsense that men carried on with. Now, I began to understand that uneasy feeling I'd always had. In happy times, the feeling was barely there. At other times it was so strong as to cause me bewilderment and anger. It was the feeling of being run from outside myself, like one of those battery-operated toys. My country, my life, even my own head were at the mercy of others. Those others were men. My feeling of always being shoved aside was a response to political reality.

At that stage Máirín de Burca's definition of occupied country had to do with Irish nationalism. For me, turned on to an acceptance of my political awareness by her remark, it pretty soon came to mean what it will always mean for me. Women live in occupied country. Does it matter much to a woman if her "own" men are running her life, or someone else's men? Has a country's freedom ever freed its women? Can a woman feel patriotic when all governments treat her as an unequal citizen and guarantee her only inferior status?

It was to take years before I had the courage to tell Máirín de Burca what I thought, that neither capitalism or socialism served women. Capitalists treat us as property. Socialists treat us like men. But by then Máirín had come to realise that socialist men were not basically more concerned about women's lives than any other group of men. She had become more feminist than pro-woman socialist, living with me in occupied country.

What fired Máirín de Burca into being a political activist was a book she read when she was thirteen years old. She had borrowed it from the children's library where she lived in Newbridge. It was called *The Young Irelanders*, by T.D. O'Sullivan, and she took it because it was the thickest book on the shelf and in the days before television, would last the longest.The book decided her to join Sinn Féin, but the organisation would not accept her until she was sixteen. Her craze for politics lasted for twenty-three years.

For me, at any rate, Máirín de Burca, the revolutionary of the early 'seventies, stands convicted of the worst her accusers said she might do. Thank heavens. She politicised me by her words and her example. I had been a "normal" woman who had worn my boredom with political discussion as a badge of femininity in male company.

As the Irish women's movement became more and more active, the yells of "lesbians", "malcontents" "unfeminine", "man-haters", were balanced with warnings to us, innocent Irish women, against being corrupted by the likes of de Burca, a "lefty revolutionary and trouble-maker." The revolutionaries, we were told, had infiltrated the group to corrupt us with socialist and nationalist motives. The latter, in those days, were not nearly as threatening as they would be today.

I think the "lefties" succeeded, to a degree at any rate, because they were politically alive. It was this aliveness that attracted. Máirín's fearless vitality would have drawn me had she merely been arranging flowers. At first I viewed her as an odd bod, with her sensible appearance, always going or coming, it seemed, from some demonstration, sit-in or march. Her unselfconscious dedication to changing the world was impressive. I remember going through an agonising period of social idealism at home as a girl, to be jeered out of it by family remarks. She had stayed her course. She was content in her work as a political activist. She had won status for herself, a woman, in her political party, and was joint secretary. And yet in giving herself so completely to a cause outside what I thought should be her human needs, she puzzled me. She seemed somehow to be suspended, a sleeping beauty, not bothering with past or present, yet obsessed with the future. Everything for Máirín seemed to be in the future. She would awaken after the revolution. She was into doing, always doing, rather than being and was incapable of wasting a minute.

She lived with her cats in a flat of her own. She took great pleasure in living on her own. As other little girls might dream of grown-up dresses, romance and marriage, Máirín had dreamed of revolution and of living alone in her own place. I could not imagine Máirín agonising over some private hurt or tossing wakefully in her bed at night. Her unwillingness to accept trauma into her life, even ours, made her appear cold on occasion. She was caring of the whole world, friendly, cheerful. I tried to get close to her because I liked her and she excited me, but she didn't even notice. She was very busy.

Quite simply, I suppose, she had recognised her vocation and was fulfilled by it. Her income seemed frugal enough, her work hard, her needs simple.

Máirín de Burca was born in Dublin and raised in Chicago. She was eight years old when her mother, Mary Margaret Farrell, a farmer's daughter, brought her brother and herself home to Kildare. Her father followed three years later. She went to school at a Sacred Heart Convent and remembers being "as free as a bird" until she left. The freedom was due to her not having to learn Irish or write exams, because her education had started in America. She went to work in a job at fourteen, having developed no other ambition than to be a Sinn Féiner.

Máirín has always had a fierce thing about security. She cannot understand how it came to mean so much to her, given that the family were always financially secure, her father being the sort of man who handed up his carpenter's pay packet unopened. They never knew want. But Máirín seems to have lost out on parental love or demonstrated affection. When her father died, in recent years, Máirín realised that she had never got to know him. She didn't really have a clue what sort of person he was. He was a moody man, but she knew nothing of his hopes or fears, had never met the man. The children were sent to bed before he came home from work, and he would take them for a drive on Sundays. She cannot remember ever having a conversation with him. She did not hit it off with her mother. Máirín remembers her mother, also dead, as someone she emotionally defended herself against when she was a child. She was possessively fixated on her son but appears to have rejected her daughter. As Máirín became increasingly conscious of feminism, she grew to understand her mother more. "I think she must have been unhappy without, perhaps, even knowing it or knowing why herself." She was the sort of woman who might have been better off without children and in later life remarks she made led Máirín to believe that her mother had felt caged and bored. Who knows what her dreams and ambitions might have been? Whatever they were, Mrs. de Burca never shared them with her daughter. Nor did it work the other way round. Máirín kept her thoughts to herself. As she spoke about the relationship, it occurred to me that perhaps the child had been a chip off the mother. Maybe the two women had more in common than they knew. Often, the child who demands the least, gets the least.

A result of her lonely childhood is probably her total self-sufficiency and ability to tackle the world as a loner. Her way of reaching out, of giving affection, is to be concerned about everybody and she manages the human need to give in that way. Her idealism, although she is a concretely practical person, she got from history books in the same way as other girls get romantic notions from love stories and pulp magazines. It is rare to meet a person who does not have great respect for Máirín, who does not mention her integrity, her political incorruptibility, but rare also to meet anybody who has got personally very close to her. The modern psychologists would probably see this as a gap in her personality, and want to psychoanalyse her into "forming close relationships", but I think they'd be completely wrong. If she had opted for religion instead of politics, her almost mystical detachment from individual involvements would be better understood. Celibacy, we are told, is a vocation because it frees the religious person to devote themselves unselfishly to everyone, not tie themselves down selfishly to one small group. Perhaps the same is true of politics and revolution.

Máirín left home forever when she was eighteen years old. She has lived alone with her cats ever since. When she was a small child in Chicago in the middle of the war, there was a shop at the corner owned by a German. She remembers him having a pretty rough time during the war. The people stopped coming into his shop, says Máirín, and he was a lovely old man and felt terrible about it. She was passing a vacant lot beside his shop one sunny day and: "There were two kittens playing on a drainpipe and one of them would go in and the other one would pounce at it when it came out, then the other one would come out and pounce. They were beautiful. I had never seen kittens before and I stood for what must have been an hour watching these kittens playing. That was it as far as I was concerned. I was going to have cats. I didn't have one until we came home to Ireland. My mother promised me that when we came home to live in the country, we'd have a cat. I don't suppose I've ever been very long without cats ever since."

Since leaving active politics, Máirín de Burca has built up a fine career as a journalist, and is buying her own home, a lifelong ambition. And yet, she says, "I am oppressed. I am oppressed by every other woman's oppression for starters. Women are still paid less than men, given the dreadful jobs, the grinding, stupid jobs, and even though that doesn't affect me personally, I'm brought down by it. And then we come back to social attitudes, you see. I'm a journalist, I'm buying my own house, I've got a loan from the bank. But the social attitudes that consider me inferior because I am a woman affect me. I feel that very strongly."

Having a need for security, Máirín used to think it would be worth getting married for that reason. Unable to account for what she describes as her "fetish" for security, she used to feel that a married woman was secure: "That's nonsense, because a poor married woman, if her husband dies and the income is wiped out, has no security at all and probably has three or four kids on top of that. I used to feel that marriage might be worth it for the security it gave you. You needn't be afraid for the future. It's daft."

Sometimes a minus can turn into a plus, and Máirín sees growing up without the sexual urges which can tie people in knots as "luck". "I might have been the sort of person that had a tremendous sexual need and drive and still have been the sort of person I am, not being able to live with another human being. Imagine that for a terrible contradiction, if you like. I couldn't live with people and I had no sexual need to live with people, which was really the ideal if you work it out."

"Have you ever wondered what all the fuss is about sex?"

"I know what all the fuss is about. Enough people go on about it and nobody says it is unpleasant except people who have been raped or had it against their will. I think that people who have sex, really against their will, are people who have been badly educated or who have had traumatic experiences as children or like poor unfortunate women in the eighteenth century who were terrified of becoming pregnant anyway. To them it was appalling because it might mean another mouth to feed."

"But you've never been interested in trying sex?"

"No. I might have tried if it didn't mean getting close to somebody else. I have never wanted to be close to another human being, not that close, because that would mean being involved. There was no way I was going to be involved on that level with anybody."

In the same vein, she says she didn't want children and would never have had them if she had married. She was never educated into babies, she says, being the baby of the family herself without other babies around. "Children would destroy my nicely organised little life. It's a selfish attitude, I suppose, but there's no way I can change."

And yet de Burca cares, practically, about children more than a lot of people who rear them. She has always spoken fiercely about the Irish state's failure to cherish all the children of the land equally as it promises to do in the Constitution. She has also referred to the family as a destructive unit in which children are at risk. She shivers visibly when she talks of the vulnerability of children and their being so much at the mercy of adults in the privacy of the home.

A tale of her own childhood, gleaned during the years I have known her, is of Máirín being told to sit on a chair when she was misbehaving. She could have been only a toddler at the time and as she sat her mother spoke to a friend on the telephone: "I can't stand Máirín anymore. She's too bold, you can come and take her if you like. You will? OK?" And then Mrs. de Burca would put down the 'phone and tell Máirín: "You sit there. So-and-So is coming to collect you."

Since I am among the many mothers who suffer remorse for similar isolated acts of cruelty to my children, I do not believe that the woman was such a demon in the context of her circumstances and the day-to-day, endless battle with house and child-rearing. Still, this little charade obviously had a devastating effect on a small girl. Máirín says she remembers sitting on the chair, sitting and sitting, waiting to be taken away, forever.

She has observed many other families and feels that for the sake of the children, there is a better way than the nuclear family yet to be found. "I think that if a married couple tear each other to pieces, well, they are adults and they can deal with it as adults deal with each other. If they tear the children to pieces, there is nothing the child can do, the child is totally vulnerable, totally at their mercy. I honestly think that it is a very rare family in which the child is not torn apart in some way, either used as a football between the parents or used for the parental ambitions. Children are used in all sorts of ways simply because they are so helpless. I don't know what the ideal set-up for rearing children would be. It may be the extended unit. It may be a concept nobody has even thought of yet. I object to people thinking you are being anti-religious when you say that the family unit is a structure that should be destroyed or should be wound up, because I don't think it has anything to do with religion at all. I see it purely from the point of view of the child."

"Oppressive" is the word Máirín uses to describe the Irishwoman's condition in marriage. She doesn't see that the Women's Movement in Ireland has had much effect on women rearing children in marriage. Certainly she thinks that there are women who now wouldn't dream of giving up their work, but who would have been into the kitchen sink thing had it not been for the consciousness-raising of the women's movement. But marriage, in the majority of cases, says Máirín, is still a sacrifice on the part of the woman.

"But in America," I remind her, "where the women's movement has gone further than in most countries, women are still getting married and re-marrying."

"I think in America," says Máirín, "the problem is extreme social pressure. Every American soap opera, every American TV programme, most American films, all assume that marriage is the inevitable state for a woman. That affects feminists too. It is just battered at them. I think that is why in America, where you have such a strong feminist movement on the one hand, you still have a great dedication to the traditional wedding, 2.5 children or whatever. It can, and does, go hand in hand."

Nine out of ten second marriages in America last, says Máirín. It seems obvious to her that if people marry young, by the time they reach thirty they want something else in a partner. They change in their needs. The ideal situation is for people to marry at least twice, if not three times: "If this became an accepted social fact it would be easier to deal with. The way it is, people marrying once and staying married all their lives, causes society to crack up when it doesn't work out. We don't know what to do with the children, who will have custody, who will do this, that and the other, and what will we do with the marital home. If society accepted that more than one marriage was the norm we'd have to devise a structure that would accommodate two or three marriages that wouldn't tear the children apart or make for a very nasty relationship between the two people separating. It would be an accepted thing that they got divorced when they matured or moved on to the next stage."

Máirín believes that if men bore babies, there would be nothing to debate about abortion. It would be automatic.

"I wouldn't be capable of saying to a woman 'you must bear this child whether you want to or not', because it isn't like telling her to put up with a headache today and it will be gone tomorrow, I think it is appalling cruelty to say that to a woman. I believe that in nine out of ten cases only the woman has the right to choose. The man would only have a say if he stood by the woman and talked it out with her on an intelligent adult level, about her needs. I don't think all this rubbish about murder would come into it if men had babies. I don't say that lots of women aren't against abortion, but mostly it's men. Men saying: 'How dare you not want my baby' or 'how dare you not want his baby'."

I mention my conflict with the fact that people who decide on abortion are already born.

"A lot of them wouldn't give a shit if they hadn't been. I cannot understand this extraordinary urge to fill every square inch of earth with people. I know God said to fill the earth or something ..."

" 'Go forth and multiply' is what He said."

"Well, I don't think that should be taken literally!"

Other political people in the founder group of women's liberation said things like "so and so is utterly middle-class" and therefore wiped her out of mind and existence. Máirín says she never felt like that. She had been used to a narrow group of people in Sinn Féin. Suddenly she had this big wide circle and found it interesting because, for the first time, she was hearing all sorts of different points of view, from all sorts of different backgrounds, walks of life, people who wouldn't have stood Sinn Féin for two minutes, people who didn't mind it, people who supported it. She felt a comradely feeling with almost all of the women. She says, too, that she loved the discussions at the big general meeting.

I had always thought Máirín missed the consciousness-raising sessions because she disapproved of that kind of subjective indulgence. Instead, it was because she came straight from her Sinn Féin meeting to our meeting. Come ten o'clock, she found she was sick with hunger, so she would skip consciousness-raising and go down and have her tea. "I missed some of the most interesting discussions. I was furious when people would come down and tell me what had gone on. For instance there was one when they discussed what was their impression when they saw their first penis ..."

"What was your impression?"

"It didn't mean a thing to me. I was a child and it was just part of my brother's anatomy. I've seen them on statues and things. I must be the only woman of my acquaintance who never met a flasher or anything like that. Nobody ever tried to frighten me out of my wits. I remember you burst into tears over the penis meeting. What was that about?"

I told her about my experience with the baby-sitter, who punished me for playing a game that he'd started, and the trauma of reliving that three-year-old child's experience in front of a group of grown-up women.

There were always a lot of traumas, it seems to Máirín. She recalls a good left-wing boy-friend of one of the women, pretending to be liberal, who actually loathed her involvement with women. Máirín was chatting to her for ages this night, when yer man came in and stood looking at her for a few minutes and then picked up his haversack and hurled it across the room at her. Máirín remembers thinking "so much for supportive men". The woman was mortified, so many of the women being there, having adjourned from the meeting upstairs. We didn't see too much of her after that.

Then there was an incident with Nell McCafferty. Máirín walked into the room to find forty women in an atmosphere you could cut with a knife. Nuala Fennell was stormy-faced in the corner and Nell's mascara was in streaks down her face. Nell, with mascara? Anyway, that's how Máirín remembers it. Nell was crying and drinking from a bottle of wine, the way they do in films when it all pours down your chin.

"I just watched and watched knowing that Nell was in

the middle of something, and I remember Nuala doing her bit about I'm not oppressed, I'm in the movement to help other women who are oppressed, I'm happily married, I love my children, I love my husband. Anyway, Nell turned round, as only Nell can do, and looked her up and down as only Nell can look you up and down and in her Northern accent said 'Oh yeh, and when was the last time you fucked your husband?' "

The whole place exploded in uproar. Máirín did her best to cope, pouring sympathetic cups of tea down the inconsolable Nell, but drew the line at bringing her home. Sympathy and comfort, sisterhood even, must be kept out in the open:

"I didn't want the trauma in my flat. I do have this terrible thing about relationships. I can't bring that sort of thing home. I could deal with it in the office, I will deal with it on the street, as I have done. I will go all day rampaging up and down a street in a demonstration or anything like that, but I will not bring it home with me. No way can I do that. There always has to be my quiet, peaceful flat at the back."

For ages, Máirín de Burca felt she didn't want to go public with Women's Liberation until we'd had about three years' gestation period. At the time she saw the movement as an extension of her other activities. As well as being secretary of Sinn Féin, she was also involved in the organisation's paper. She was in the Housing Action Committee and had squatted in Hume Street when buildings there were being torn down. She was in the Anti-Apartheid movement and the Campaign against the Forcible Entry Bill and very involved with political prisoners and the national question. To the forefront was what was happening in Northern Ireland in 1968/9. Before there was a real meeting at all, either in Mary Maher's or Mary Kenny's, Máirín had met with Margaret Gaj and Mary Maher in Bewley's and discussed the condition of women in Ireland.

Many people were puzzled as to how housing and the Forcible Entry Bill, for instance, were feminist issues.

Máirín was adamant about housing. If women stayed home and had large families, how could housing conditions not be a main issue, she argued. She won her point.

The Forcible Entry Bill grew out of the housing situation. Sinn Féin had been putting squatters into empty property and the Forcible Entry bill was brought in to stop this, so that squatters could be arrested. I well remember trying to help one of the Sinn Féin squatters during that time. Let's call her Mrs. Mooney. I collected money for her through my column in the *Sunday Independent* and spent weeks and weeks bringing her groceries and food for the children. I never did succeed in sorting out the woman's situation. Dublin Corporation had files and files dealing with her housing problem. It had got to the stage that other Corporation tenants did not wish to live next door to this family. It took ages for me to realise that she was a psychopathic liar who made up a script as she went along, was manipulative, thoroughly dishonest and an awful sneak. She accused her husband of being a male prostitute and of renting her out for prostitution. Not even after she had complained to the editor that I was keeping the money intended for her did I give up on Mrs. Mooney. Máirín, though, could manage her fine. The family, no matter how anti-social, needed a house, and Sinn Féin had put them squatting. Eventually, feeling that only a squad of experts working full-time for at least a couple of years could sort out the Mooneys with their variety of problems, I abandoned the family and felt guilty. Through Máirín's eyes I could see myself as a silly do-gooder who deserved the lesson.

Máirín went to jail with Marie McMahon in 1971, charged with an offence under the Diplomatic Immunity Act, because they were in a demonstration at the American Embassy about the Vietnam War. Cow's blood was poured on the steps, and the US flag was burned. The demonstration coincided with a big mobilisation in America on the same day, 24 April 1971. Thirteen people took part and they could have got away, but decided that they would not. In their innocence they decided to stay and answer for what they had done. Four of them went to prison for three months.

Until that time, Máirín de Burca had been a leading Sinn Féin proponent of the political status theory. She had spoken on numerous platforms about political status. She had decided that should she ever go to prison she would claim political status, but reality quickly changed her view of that.

She had spent the previous twelve months with the Women's Liberation Movement, so that her feminism was at a fairly high level. Suddenly she realised that women in prison were her natural colleagues in the feminist struggle. She found them pathetic, sad and even happy, but a cross-section of women. "You always asked each other what you were in for and having done that you got it out of the way, it was never referred to again. You then got on the level of just being colleagues in a particular, very oppressive, unpleasant, desperate situation. There was this tremendous bond. I'd have almost died for any of the girls there, although I didn't know them from Adam and they didn't know me. They wanted to go on a hunger strike once because of something that happened to us and not because they would have been with us in what we'd done. I would have done the same for them."

Máirín says that from then on there was no cutting one-self off and demanding special status because you weren't a criminal. It just wasn't on and she stopped seeing the point of it forever more, particularly in relation to feminists. Now she believes that most prisoners are political. There is a certain section of the population, a tiny, tiny section, who are evil people, bad people who would hurt others at the drop of a hat without it costing them a thought, but they are a terribly tiny minority. The vast majority of people in prison are there for social reasons, she feels now. Like the vast majority of psychiatric patients, she adds.

Prison affected Máirín very deeply. Marie McMahon once said that Máirín seemed to melt in prison. She cried, and couldn't cope with being locked up and ordered around. A pacifist, never guilty of a violent action despite all her verbal protests, de Burca was shocked by the treatment they received. She recalls it as the most serious thing that had ever happened to her in her life. She had been a very free person, no responsibilities, no family, used to doing what she wanted, when she wanted. Suddenly she found herself locked up all day and all night, locked behind stone walls. She says it still affects her, and uses the word "affect" where another might say "hurt".

On another occasion, Mary Anderson and she were arrested when the founder group stormed the Dáil in protest against the Forcible Entry Bill. I was near Máirín when she was lifted — and also close to one of the more ladylike among the sisterhood, who said haughtily to the policeman: "Don't you dare touch me, I'm a doctor's wife!"

The night the Forcible Entry Bill was being passed, the opposition tried to stone-wall it a bit; the government decided they'd put a guillotine on it and it was passed very quickly. We were all waiting for the Ministers to come out in their state cars and we were going to shout at them. "Can you imagine," asks Máirín, "that was all we were going to do? When you think of things that happened to people later on, with killings and murderings and bombings, we were ferociously innocent. We were actually going to shout at them, that was all we were going to do. If the Minister had got out of his car and stood in front of us, we would have been flummoxed."

In any case, when the crowd of women were seen at the gate, the drivers drove out with the cars and the Ministers went out some other way and met them. So we found ourselves yelling at empty cars.

Mary and Máirín were arrested. I remember Máirín looking calm and the police speaking respectfully to her and Anderson purple with rage and struggling. And that was the beginning of the Juries Act, because the women opted for a trial by jury, and only then realised that a jury would consist of twelve property-owning men. They had been charged with breach of the peace. Máirín asked Senator

Mary Robinson how they could make a protest in court about being tried by twelve property-owning men without being sent down for contempt and she said: "You can't really make a protest in court without being sent down for contempt, but what you could do is take a Constitutional action, because I believe that the Juries Act is, in fact, unconstitutional." After a bit of delicate hovering between the three of them it was agreed that she would take the case, knowing full well that neither would be able to pay her, and that they could not afford to lose, because costs would be awarded against them.

They did not lose. Jury service in Ireland is now open to anyone over eighteen who is on the register of electors. Barristers complained subsequently that compensation for injuries, which was pretty high, slumped alarmingly when the new Juries Act came into operation. Women were not used to large sums of money, says Máirín, and giving damages that *they* thought were massive, gave less than had been given before. No businessman would have looked twice at the amounts given by women, and the lawyers were furious about it.

Máirín left Sinn Féin in July of 1977. The last eight years of her involvement with the party had been the busiest, and she felt physically tired. If disillusion with the masculine orientation of the party was part of the tiredness, she never publicly stated this. Long before, she had started loosening herself from the fallacy that under social- ism the women's struggle would be over. She still believes that under socialism the legal oppression of women would be ended. There would be equal pay, equal training, crêches and nursery schools, but now she also sees that this would not mean the amelioration of women's conditions unless social attitudes changed. Now she recognises that women have to organise themselves to go beyond socialism, to change social attitudes. Some elements in Sinn Féin had always resisted Máirín's involvement with what they called bourgeois liberal feminist issues such as contraception. Contraception was bourgeois because it wasn't an economic issue. She tried to point out that it wasn't any of those things because women couldn't go back to work unless there were freely available contraceptives.

"It was once seriously suggested to me by a party member that the party should forget about women who weren't at work, because they were not organised workers, they weren't part of the industrial workforce and they were therefore a pain in the ass and a waste of time." Her views on divorce and the value of women's work in the home met with similar attitudes. Through it all, Máirín decided that socialism was not enough. She became a feminist, as distinct from having been a pro-woman socialist.

She began to say things which could be quite unpopular in a socialist organisation, for instance, she said that there might come a time when it would be far more important to attend your feminist meeting than to attend a Sinn Féin party meeting. She admits she began to blame men more for women's oppression and says now she has never met a true male feminist. She believes that men's attitudes to women basically end up with self-interest. "I get a bit pissed off when men tell me that basically they understand the women's struggle. They don't, and I'd just as soon they wouldn't say it."

Máirín sees women, because of social attitudes, "freed" to do two jobs instead of one. Men are not asked to be co-workers inside the home. She remembers a visitor from Poland, a socialist state, being horrified to discover that Mrs. Gaj's sons washed their socks. The visitor had one child, the child was in a crêche, she worked all day, had her own money, and to us was madly liberated. And yet, in her broken English, she managed to say that men didn't wash socks. She would have died, says Máirín, to defend her right to all the benefits she had in Poland, but her social attitude was that men didn't wash their own socks.

Máirín's departure from Sinn Féin followed an eight-week speaking tour of America. She had looked forward to it as a holiday because in eight years she hadn't had one. The trip was a terrible job of work and she came back in bits, determined to leave it all.

She got a job cleaning offices before she left the party,

because, typically, she wouldn't leave without any income at all. Between the work and welfare, she was in receipt of £18 a week. After seven months, she got a job in the Irish Post Office Engineering Union as a typist. She enjoyed working in an all-female office.

Before that, Máirín was registered with five employment agencies. Four of them didn't bother on her behalf, thinking her a hopeless case for employment in Ireland. In the fifth, a young woman from Liverpool tried, and discovered the Irish thing about people and politics. Telephones were banged down, excuses made, jobs always filled. The woman dug her heels in and said: "I'm going to get you a job if it kills me!" She put Máirín's name down with one other person who was either unable to spell or to type, they forget which. And she said: "If you don't get this job we'll know it's discrimination and we'll take it further." Máirín got the job. To be fair to Séamus de Paor, says Máirín, he never hesitated to employ her, even though there was pressure to keep her out.

She had journalistic experience and had tried for jobs on papers. She got odd bits of free-lancing, but not enough to keep body and soul together. She took anything, even writing in *Social and Personal*, which seemed an unlikely place to find her name. Eventually, after the third try, she landed a job with *Hibernia* and continued into *The Sunday Tribune* when the former paper died.

No longer an activist, Máirín de Burca plunged into print in the *Irish Times* in the winter of 1980 in opposition to Nell McCafferty's claim that the Provisional IRA women on the dirty protest in Armagh Jail were a feminist issue. This issue seemed to tear Irish feminists apart. Those against said that it could not be a feminist issue, since the actions of these women were directed by male politics and resulted in death and heartbreak to other "sisters" in the North. Besides, it was repeatedly asked would the women in Armagh jail even know what the word "feminist" meant?

Probably not, replied McCafferty, weren't the Armagh women only "wee wains" when the troubles began, and what had they had the time or opportunity for save the battle on their door-steps? The rising of the women *was* the rising of the race, claimed the Derrywoman who wrote *The Armagh Women*. Máirín de Burca, in reply to the Armagh women as a feminist issue, claimed that feminism should provide no shelter for élitism. Somewhere along the line some man discovered, Máirín pointed out acidly, that a woman could pull the trigger and stop a bullet every bit as efficiently as a man. "Some of the younger ones needed a thin version of feminist jargon mixed with the Mother of Ireland stuff to put them in the right frame of mind, but that was no problem, just as it had been no problem to incorporate the more respectable bits of Marx and Lenin in with Padraig Pearse to quieten the other lot. Women were just as good at going to prison as men, too, and could be relied upon to parrot the prison protests as efficiently as they had done the terrorism outside. They had not been encouraged to question the basis of this whole physical force merry-go-round so why would they suddenly discover their common sisterhood with other women prisoners?" asked Máirín, in a page of replies to Nell McCafferty in the *Irish Times*. "Our male masters," said Máirín, "had told us that we could only be freed by death and destruction, so we obediently shot and bombed and helped them to shoot and bomb. All of that is called the struggle against imperialism and it's blessed by apostolic succession, with Maud Gonne and the Green Countess thrown in for those who baulk at an all male pantheon."

The regrettable thing, as Máirín points out, is that the Founder's Group of Women's Liberation broke up before nationalism became the big thing that it has subsequently become. Because of one thing and another, it was never subjected to the cold light of feminist examination. Have women an affinity with nationalism? asks Máirín. She does not believe that they have, necessarily. Anyway, it has never been put under the feminist microscope. Now there are groups such as the 32-County Women's Liberation, Women Against Imperialism, Women Fighting for the Armagh Twenty-Five. Máirín would like a chance to discuss it in a cool atmosphere. Are these women taking a male-dominated ideology, adopting it whole, not even saying: "Well, yes, that part of nationalism doesn't conflict with feminist ideals," or are they swallowing the lot, hook, line and sinker?

"I have actually heard women saying that the most important feminist demand in the North is the end of oppression. Feminist demand? Jesus Christ! Women say that because they first heard men saying it. Men have invented our slogans, they've designed our uniforms, they've handed us guns. We should be asking if this is what feminists should be doing. It is the same with the political prisoners thing. Nobody has sat down and said: 'is this a feminist thing to be doing, demanding separate status from other women?' "

Máirín de Burca lives less in the past these days. Her three-roomed artisan dwelling house was described as "middle-class" in a magazine feature by Nuala Fennell in which the latter even presented the colour of Máirín's lavatory paper as evidence of the revolutionary having come to heel, joined up with the comfort of the status quo: "It's a bit much to have one's loo paper taken down and used in evidence," says Máirín. "Apparently it matched the walls."

Máirín has won for herself the basic rights for which she fought on behalf of others, a job and a home. In going beyond that, she expresses the feminist goal of self-definition. She has pulled the little house around her like a blanket, adapting it to suit the realities of her life and her conscience, as she has done with ideologies.

11
NELL

"Who made the world?" Nell McCafferty will ask me suddenly when I'm in the down mood she hates.

"We did, Nell," I say on cue, in tender joke. Well, we did try to change the shape of our lives, to make a world in which women could live. We tried ...

Who made the world is surely a question I was asked and answered every day of my childhood. "God made the world." Nell doesn't remember being asked that. She was struck by it when Derryman Eamonn McCann, author and *Sunday World* journalist, repeated it to her one day, saying it had been part of his Catholic education. Nell doesn't think she was ever asked that as a child in Derry. Maybe it was only taught to boys? In any case, now she believes that those first Irishwomen to join in the Irish Women's Liberation Movement were taking over at some place where God left off. Not that Nell would give God credit for everything up until then.

"Maybe you mean we women are taking over from the eighth or ninth day?" I ask Nell.

"Naw," she says, "the world was incomplete in our lives because women didn't figure, but now women are shaping their world and it is wonderful. I think what we did was wonderful. Not much? Measured against what? It wasn't just us. Obviously women were ready and there were other forces at work, but we are the ones who stood up and I feel terrific about that. It gave me a great understanding about how you make history."

The suggestion that we are all forgotten or considered as rearguard freaks makes Nell laugh out in joy: "I was there," she says, "I know I took part. I know what I did."

Nell McCafferty was born in one of Derry's little red-brick terrace houses which climb either side of the hill streets in the Bogside. In the rest of the country Nell may be a star, loved or disliked for her Dickensian insight and her wicked wit, author, journalist, broadcaster, radical feminist, but there on Richmond Street, Nell is just "our Nell" home from Dublin. Mothers of the Bogside remember "our Nell" as "always just like one of the wee lads playing outside. One of the McCafferty girls, but more like a boy. A grand wee wain."

Nell still looks like a tousled urchin, except for the wide blue eyes that could only be a woman's, the breasts on the stocky little body. Nell was once refused admission to a Dublin nightclub because of her appearance: "I suppose they thought my hair unkempt and my breasts unruly," Nell told me.

"Womanly" describes Nell. She's earthy, ripe in herself. Her charity surprised me before I discovered her warmth and her hungry way of listening. Anyone can stop her in the street and tell their life's story and she'll stand there listening, looking up intently until the rain sends them both into a doorway or a pub. Man, woman or child, Nell empathises with the victim. She is a victim of victims, not because of what they ask of her, but because of what she feels.

It was that empathy which created Nell's column "In The Eyes Of The Law", later compiled as a book, in the *Irish Times*. How many journalists before Nell had sat in the Districts Court or the Children's Courts reporting the process of law as it applied to the poor, the helpless and the hapless, as if it made sense? Which one of us ever dreamed of putting the law, the bench, society on trial? Nell *was* that mother trying to go bail for her son when she wrote:

A modest middle-aged woman entered the witness

box of Dublin District Court 6 to go bail for her son.

"What is your occupation?" the Justice asked her. "Housewife", she named the condition that has been hymned in praise by church and state.

Where would she get £100 if the defendant did not appear to answer charges, the Justice asked.

"I have me husband's wages. And then I do a bit of cleaning work meself," the woman said.

"How much do you earn a week?" the Justice asked.

"Twenty pounds," she replied.

"I can't accept you. I'm refusing you." The Justice rejected this mother, this cleaning woman, this wife. Her lifetime's work of rearing children and scrubbing office floors and keeping a marriage together was not sufficient to buy her son's freedom, while awaiting trial."

I didn't really get to know Nell until I visited Lily, her mother, in 1976 when Nell was off in America, free as a bird and writing home. Nell, self-conscious in her freedom and conscious of home, the heart of Britain's Irish problem, felt guilty. We sat, Lily and I, having our tea under the room in which all six McCafferty children were born. Nell had written from a hot stoop in New Orleans. It was a letter of sisterhood to a mother. Nell, as she wrote from what she was experiencing as paradise, was also Lily getting the letter in the place Nell knows and loves so well. "I wish you could have this, Ma," she said in half-a-dozen different ways, "you deserve it." And that was of its essence, an exquisite empathy with another woman's life. It was as if Nell was in the room with us, in Lily's past, and at the same time struggling with a separation that left one the loser and the other unable to accept her gain.

Nell was especially close to Lily, possibly because as a child she suffered from rheumatic fever and was away from school half the year. "She always took me out shopping during the week when I was in my 'teens and I used to love it, because we went around all the shops

paying her debts and I knew what her debts were and I saw
her debts book. I'm not sure if the others did. And we
used to feel proud to strike another shilling off Cavendish's
and that, and what I couldn't understand is, how, if we
were so broke, we could afford to go across the road to
Stephenson's. It's a sort of a tea shop and we'd go in and
have a cup of tea and a lemon pancake each. And I knew
the cost of that. And we'd get the bus home. And I was
perfectly aware that the cost of that would have paid off
Cavendish's for another week. But we did it. And it was
lovely. Except that we always had to be home by six
because my father had to have his dinner on the table
when he got home. I was raging about that and I knew she
was raging too."

It was from her father Nell remembers first becoming
aware of the power of a word. It was at intermediate
school and she was doing an essay on a postman during
lunch-time. Her father and she did it together and talked
about the postman and her father said he wore a blue serge
suit. "I was impressed by the word 'serge'. It was a
concrete word for describing something. I was intrigued by
the way it helped to paint the picture of the postman."

Nell's father was a religious man who told her once: "If
you question your faith too much, you'll lose it," and it
was from him she learned to question. He didn't drink and
was considered a "wee gentleman" because he always wore
a hat. Nell now understands him as a frustrated intellectual.
She describes him as the "original patriarch in the corner",
providing for everybody but not knowing how to share the
power. He was as dead set against socialism as he was
against sex, she recalls, although he used to say you should
always pay your debts and the labourer must be paid his
wages.

Derry was a port in those days and Nell's father worked
for the British Admiralty as a store-house clerk. She could
never understand what her father did for a living: "I
remember he used to have to climb up on top of the oil
tanks and dip and come home smelling of oil. I just
couldn't understand all the figures he was using. He

explained the job to me often and I'd have to say: 'I don't know what you're talking about, Da.' And he used to come home at six every evening on his bike and we'd be at the end of the row, me and Hugh and Paddy, and he'd get off his bike and take us up on the bar and the saddle home. Why'd he change, the bastard?"

Mr. McCafferty changed when the youngsters started having dates. "He became aware we were all sexually active human beings and it blew his mind." Now he wanted them all home at a certain time every night. From the age of six until about thirteen Nell had been free every night with her friend Joe and it didn't matter to her father and mother that Joe was "different". "I always knew there was something different about Joe. He had a mother who was kind of simple, she used to always give us bread and jam and we'd run in and out of her house. I had a feeling that Joe didn't have as much money as we did, I knew he was somehow different. It was only years later I discovered that he was what they call illegitimate and Joe was considered odd by everybody else because he didn't go to school. But that's the way it was then. He didn't go to school because his mother wasn't capable or it didn't matter or he was a child without a parent. The other kids thought Joe was stupid. We spent all our time together. We used to sit up on the back wall of people's houses and look in, at night, and watch them have fights or talk or eat or we used to go through the fields at night. We spent a lot of time out at night together. It was very peaceful walking around the town. It was Joe and me for about seven years and then I dropped him."

Nell arrived at the age when with the other McCaffertys she was busting to get out to a céilí and they'd have to rush to get home. Their father would be waiting: "Where were you? You're late, what were you doing?" "I knew what he meant, but there was no way I could say: 'listen, I wasn't doing it', or 'I know what you're talking about, but nothing could be further from my mind'. And he was so worried all the time. My mother would say, 'Jimmy, leave them alone.' And my eldest sister Muireanna came in for the worst of it. Maybe because she was the first and she was gorgeous. She jived, she was into the Bill Haley thing, she wore the make-up and she was lively. Boys used to come and serenade her, five at a time with guitars in our front room. It was the foreign sailors that worried all the parents in Derry. They were golden-skinned, with golden money, and the Derry boys by comparison were pimply, pale-faced and unemployed."

Nell was very happy as a child in Derry. She recalls wishing she could be sick for ever because her favourite nun at school gave her sticky buns every morning and was so nice to her. And Nell thought that she was happy as a result of being sick. Grammar school was a bit different. There she became aware that the daughters of the doctors and solicitors would be head girls. They were swanky, she wasn't. "I was brainy and they weren't and I knew my mother was lovely and they weren't as happy as I was, but still they were the ones that got the credits. And I remember vaguely being unhappy at the thought of bringing them home, because they'd think my house was poor. I once brought a girl home whose father owned a factory, a very nice, amiable, but ignorant man, but with a lot of money, and I said: 'Ma, this is Margaret', and we went into the sittingroom and Ma disappeared and suddenly she came back five minutes later with a swiss roll and I knew that she had gone down the back lanes to get us a swiss roll, because it was too expensive an item to have by chance, and I remember feeling terribly hurt for my mother that she had to impress this fifteen-year-old girl. I was raging." Nell's father was never unemployed, but she remembers noticing that other people went away on holiday and they never did. Years later Lily told her that her husband used to send her for a month down to Buncrana to a caravan and she went wild, she hated it. She went back to her own house. Lily always prefers her own house. And once they went to the Gaeltacht, which they weren't aware was the Gaeltacht, and Nell remembers it was awful with nobody there except themselves; the woman spoke Irish and served them fish-heads and any time they walked to the beach, which seemed to be miles away, the tide would be out and they were all miserable and came home after four days.

"We were all born in the one house," muses Nell, "I must say I like that I know where I was born. My mother says the trouble with people nowadays is they don't know where they came from."

Nell qualified as a teacher, but couldn't get a job in a Protestant school because she was a Catholic, and not being what the Catholics called a Catholic, she could not get a job in a Catholic school. It never occurred to me that Nell could be anything other than a Derry Catholic although I knew her maternal grandmother had been a Protestant: "Well there's only two reasons I can think came against me. One is that when Eamonn McCann did a skit on a Sean O'Casey play in the University, one of my lines was "Jesus, Jesus, they're robbin' the post office", and the priest said it was blasphemous to take the Lord's name in vain. The other reason was that I'd studied psychology without asking the Bishop's permission and I said I didn't know we had to ask the bishop's permission and he said I should have known. The reason, I understood, was that in Derry if you wanted to become a teacher you went over to the Bishopry and asked the Bishop for an audience and offered your services. You did not ask for a job. You offered your services, and he accepted them or not. But I didn't even kiss his ring. I refused to do that. So the Bishop let it be known that until I came and offered my services I could forget the whole thing. And I wouldn't. Years later I discovered that my mother went to the Bishop and the Monsignor and all round the town asking: 'why can't our Nell get a job?' And another reason they gave was 'what was I doing working on a Kibbutz?' "

Having read about kibbutzim in James Michener's book, *The Source,* Nell had to get to one. She loved it. She could see a lot of things wrong with it, but her reason for coming back was that she was going bananas picking apples. Millions of apples. She left Israel after the Yom Kippur war in 1967. She says she didn't understand it, but she enjoyed being in a war. They spent a lot of time in the trenches during that war while Israeli 'planes went in to slam the Arabs. Some of the shells fell into the trenches. The men had machine-guns and the women were given blunderbusses. The women were so terrified of what the Arabs might do to them that they arranged to shoot themselves with the ancient guns. She thought of waving her passport when the Arabs came to rape them, but never got a chance to put this to the test.

Nell recalls, with regret, being involved in victorious behaviour after the Yom Kippur war. She piled into trucks with the Jews to tour the occupied Arab territories. It was like a holiday, she recalled, they won the war and they toured all the Arab places, all the land they had conquered, and went into the houses looking for stuff. The women and children had disappeared, gone to wherever you go when you are pushed out of your country. The Arabs they met treated them civilly, Nell recalls, but on a school blackboard they found drawings of terrified Arab children and Israelis with big thick noses and blood dripping from their fangs. "I thought 'how bigotted these Arabs are'."

It wasn't until 1970, when Nell knew more about politics, that she blushed at the thought of her tour of Arab country. It was when the curfew on the Falls Road was lifted. But before it was lifted, Brookeborough was taken by an army chief around the conquered territory. Nell's mother, watching the television, swore at him. "And I watched it and I thought how dare he ride around the Catholic area looking at them all penned in and frightened, so triumphant? I'd done the same after the Six Day War."

She couldn't get a job in Derry, so she went to London with everybody else. The newspapers on Fleet Street told her that if she took a job making tea and doing messages she might work her way up. And she thought "shit" and got a job in a Wimpy Bar. The job meant that she would not have to get married after all. Not that she had anybody picked out, or even suspected anyone of wanting to marry her, but in her dump of a room in London, jobless, penniless and friendless, she had decided marriage was the only thing left.

Back in Derry again, in 1968, unemployed, Nell met Eamonn McCann bouncing down the street. He lived around the corner from her, in a council house. Nell's house, she cautions with a grin, is private housing, and proud the inhabitants of Beechwood Street were the day a neighbour was refused permission from the Planning Department to open a "wee sweet-shop" in her front parlour because the street was a residential area. Nell always had a great admiration for McCann, a vital, tough and good-humoured sort of man. "You always had the sense of being alive around Eamonn", she told me once. He was unemployed, too. Nell could never again equate unemployment with being useless, a failure.

"Join the Derry Labour Party," McCann told her that day in the street, "it's great crack," and she did. Eventually, she became secretary of the DLP and gave information to all the journalists who visited Derry. They still talk about her. She didn't just give the party line. She had a flair for objective fact, she understood power, loved talking to people.

A physical coward if ever there was one, Nell had been in the thick of marches, petrol-bomb-throwing and bin-lid bush-telegraph. Non-sectarian, she was to find herself in open combat with Protestants. Hers was the party which backed the student body called "People's Democracy" which decided to march from Belfast to Derry's Burntollet knowing they'd march through Protestant territory. People said there would be a civil war as a result but the marchers' justification was that they'd merely be lancing a boil. The night before, there was a meeting of the DLP to decide whether or not they'd go on the march. Nell's mother and her Auntie Nellie went to the meeting because of Nell. They'd been to a few meetings before. Nell's mother didn't want her to march for fear she'd be killed. Finally, after many deeply emotional speeches, it came to a vote. Lily and Nellie looked at Nell and Eamonn McCann and raised their hands and the motion was passed by one vote: "So my mother and Nellie instinctively changed history, and I remember her saying afterwards: 'but to-morrow you have to sign for the dole, what are you going to do?' and I said: 'what's the dole for?' And she said: 'Jesus, you're reared'."

"We got as far as Magherafelt and on the way there was a Protestant with a hatchet behind every bush and we didn't believe they'd kill us. They'd just hurt us a wee bit. There was this small wee girl there with a crash helmet and two dirty front teeth in front saying: 'march, march, march' to keep us going. It was Bernadette Devlin and I kept thinking 'I'll march, but I'll keep well to the back because I'm not going to get killed.' At Magherafelt, which is about 20 miles from Burntollet, my heel was so blistered I couldn't march and I told a fellow, Barney Turkington, I'd have to get my heel fixed. Magherafelt was surrounded by Protestants and we couldn't get in and we were afraid to go to a doctor in case it was the wrong one and he'd kill me."

They decided to drive back to Belfast to a Catholic doctor and got back to Clogher, fifteen miles from Derry, when they heard there was going to be riots. Nell, because of her charm and gift of the gab, was sent in to find out what was happening in Derry. A lawyer, Vincent Hanna, drove her into Derry and they arrived just as Paisley's people inside the Guildhall broke up the chairs to use as weapons to fight their way out of the Hall and through the mob of "sectarian Catholics" who thought they had them trapped inside. Paisley's crowd came out of the Guildhall and swept the Catholics away. "There was," recalls Nell, "a certain amount of shame in thinking we could be beaten and we were civil rights people so we couldn't be violent. I thought it was coming near the stage of killing and we decided to go back to Clogher and tell them what had happened." On the way back the roads were blocked by the police and they were kept driving around the mountains and farms and walking down roads all night. They got to Clogher at about 10 o'clock in the morning after the march had left: "We drove after them and suddenly there was blood and students running about with their heads smashed open and bandages and clothes on the ground and what looked like Protestants to my mind and policemen laughing and I was terrified and all I could think of was my sister was on this March because she was coming from Derry to join us. I picked up one of the students, drove off with him in the back of the car and caught up with the march a mile and a half later, and they were straggling along, brave and beautiful and bleeding, singing the Internationale."

On the way again, they got trapped in a Protestant housing estate and attacked with bottles and stones. Nell was thinking what a bore it was to stand around non-violently and get killed. "I was terrified. And by that time a lot of Derry people had joined us and this seemed to us the big, revolutionary breakthrough, the working class, the dockers had arrived, my sister had arrived, we even heard John Hume was coming. I mean, this was it, John Hume, accepting the left wing. And then we were trapped in that street before the bridge with the big tall houses on either side and the Protestants were throwing stones and I remember being clever enough to say 'I'm getting in a doorway' and I beat my way through the crowd: I didn't care who I killed, I wanted to get in a doorway and be protected. I can never understand why people don't protect themselves. I stayed in the doorway and stones rained down and then finally the police who were blocking the bridge let us through and we marched across the bridge singing 'Arise you starlings from your slumber, revolt you prisoners of want.' And my sister was totally unafraid. I was crying, but my sister had known no fear. She had been trapped in a stream and some guy went over with a club with nails in it and went to beat her and some other guy rescued her, but she was genuinely not afraid ..."

"Free Derry", the Bogside taken over by its own people, has been described by Nell as "No Man's Land". She helped beat the Protestant marchers and police out of it. The Protestants were going to come marching by in a traditional parade commemorating the Siege of Derry when the Protestants, "quite rightly" as Nell told me, locked out the Catholics and King James in 1689. "What they always did wrong was to come marching through the

Catholic areas shouting: 'Catholics are pigs' and throwing them pennies. Now they were told 'don't come marching through our territory' and while the Catholics said that they were behind the scenes stacking up petrol bombs, thousands of them." If they set foot in the Bogside, they were prepared for them: "The reason we were ready to fight," says Nell, "is because *they* had the 'B' Specials, the police, and they were bigots and they were going to kill us and we'd had enough. And part of us, a wee part of us hoped they'd come in, 'cos we'd show them, us Catholics, we weren't cowards. And the Protestants came marching down the next day and unluckily, or luckily, a few of the kids threw a few stones. Maybe ten stones, but the police could not wait and put up their shields and pulled down their riot helmets and charged into the Bogside. We were delighted and within seconds we had sent word. It was like orchestrating a concerto, we sent word to the Brandywell, the Creggan, the Bogside, Shantalla, to bring in the petrol bombs. And for an hour the police were met with fire. By fuck we were ready for them. We were so organised that they couldn't break through. We didn't think about skin burning, we didn't think about killing, we were just at war and we beat them out of the Bogside. Bernadette's excuse was that we were trying to build a wall of fire in front of them. Who was she trying to kid? We were aiming at them. We were trying to burn them. I didn't think about it then. I just threw the petrol bombs. One woman was pouring petrol in, another was tearing up the blankets, another was pouring the sugar in and yet another was organising the transferral and saying 'bring back the empty bottles.' Everybody was doing that and we'd burn, burn, burn. We kept them out. And it was the policemen that acted like proper state terrorists, but the odd policeman who made the mistake of coming too far got burned. We burnt about four, but it's not true that I burned the first policeman in Derry. I'd remember that. I didn't."

Nell thought Civil Rights was over when she came to the job in Dublin. It was Mary Holland who had suggested to the *Irish Times* that they should ask Nell to write for them. They sent her a telegram requesting copy.

The best piece she did for the *Irish Times* as a free-lance was a profile of Ian Paisley. She liked him. She felt he did wish to do well by his constituents, get them houses and jobs whatever their religion: "Protestants didn't have anybody then. They were imprisoned in class relationships which had nothing to do with religion. And bigot though he be, he seemed to be strong. I was glad the Protestants had somebody strong on their side because they were being pathetic at that stage. I followed him around in the middle of the campaign in Ballymena, from 7 a.m. until around 1 o'clock and then I knocked on his door and said: 'Would you please tell me when you are coming out again, at two o'clock or three o'clock, because I'd like to eat,' and with a sandwich in his hand he said: 'I don't know when I'll be finished', and he didn't offer me a bite of his sandwich and he wouldn't ask me in and he slammed the door in my face. I followed him around all day and the *Irish Times* liked the profile and eventually asked me to come for an interview and I got the job." Lelia Doolan found a home in Dublin for Nell, and Mary Holland and Liz O'Driscoll, now Liz McManus, Councillor for the Workers' Party in Bray, and her mother gave her money against her first pay packet. "Our Nell" went off to Dublin to a good job.

Hardly anybody noticed Nell in the *Irish Times* on that big day of her life, her first day on the staff. No red carpet. Such casual treatment must have come as a disappointment to the Derrywoman coming from a place where nobody ignores anybody. Someone sent her to the women's corner and she was affronted and frightened thinking she knew nothing about fashion or babies and what would they say to her then? There was nothing for her to do so she started an article about Derry and spent a week on it and it was published. It seemed, to Nell, to go unnoticed.

"I suppose it was good or bad, but nobody in the *Irish Times* gave a shit whether I wrote or not. Now I had a job I didn't have to work. That was the thing which struck me about the world of employment, once you're in, you're in.

However badly I wrote, I had my union card and I was hired now. Sad thing, some of the journalists wrote trash. It's one of the big questions about Marxism, once you're in, you're in."

I was there the day Nell met Mary Kenny. Mary was in a glamorous mood that day with a split skirt that showed her legs and as Nell remembers: "Mary had make-up on, in that tatty way that wasn't make-up but Mary painting herself, and she came forward and she kissed me on the cheek. I don't think anybody had ever done that and if they did, I don't remember it, and she'd a glint in her eye and people didn't go on like that in Derry. She smiled and made me feel totally at home. And I wasn't ashamed. She didn't judge. Other people always did. If they didn't they were ignorant and if they weren't ignorant then they were embarrassed and whether she knew or not she was enjoying it. And maybe part of it was a chance for Mary to be outrageous, but only part. And I remember, June, you looked like a dolly-bird, but in so much as dolly-birds were teen-agers you weren't. I can remember you offering to burn your bra and me thinking 'quite right', but you can kill yourself or get sorely burnt and while you burn your bra to turn these men on, you don't have to."

I remember it differently. Someone said there had never been a bra burnt anywhere and I said it would only make sense if it was burned on the wearer. Buddhist monks were immolating themselves in Vietnam at the time. It would be worth it if people would listen, I said. Then someone said; "you do it" handing me a lighter, but when the bra caught alight Donal Foley put it out with his napkin and then plunged into his drink for fortification.

At one point I remember discussing the possibility of a feminist army, with weapons, with Mary Anderson. The scene with the bra came back when Nell mentioned it. Perhaps I'd had a drink or two, perhaps I felt like burning myself that day. Who gave me the lighter?

As for Nell, Mary Kenny brought her in, brought her out, brought her home. "From her it was acceptable, because to them *she* was normal, in those days anything went. Everything went and she was everything, it was I who was the freak. And we had great fun together because Mary was naturally so full of fun. I can remember the luxury of breakfast in bed at Mary Kenny's flat when I stayed over. It was like having a bath with you around ..."

Once in a blue moon Nell arrives at my house tired and troubled and I run the bath and put oil and bubbles in it and set towels to warm and bring her snacks with a glass of something. If she wants to talk I sit on the lavatory seat and when the water threatens to cool turn the hot tap. Or sometimes I leave her alone and just wait until she comes out refreshed, grinning, smelling like a glamorous mother carrying a baby, of scent and Johnson's Baby Lotion.

"Mary used to bring me a four-course breakfast, and I'd have it while she'd be on the 'phone organising the schedules for the day and good stories and worrying about her bank and putting her life in order, while rushing in and out of the bedroom putting on powder and perfume and tat. And off she'd go. And then things came to their natural end. It was my birthday and she knew it and she didn't come to it. I went round and threw stones at her window and she finally opened the window and said 'you're disturbing the neighbours' and I said 'fuck the neighbours'. I was in despair because I knew there was a man and I hated that a man could replace me, even a drip. Eventually Mary let me in and the next morning I put on my combat jacket and we went to Dáil Éireann where we had lunch with Michael O'Leary. Next thing I remember it was the 12th of July. It was the date Mary went off to England to a whole new life. I had this ship-to-shore call, I never had one before in my life. It was Mary saying: 'I am now looking at Dun Laoghaire lights.' And I said: 'Jesus Christ, I've had a ship-to-shore 'phone call, Mary, and it's wonderful' and she said 'sure, I know.' And my heart wasn't broken anymore. The entire ship knew she was ringing me. I was the only one she could ring."

The end of Mary Kenny and the end of the founder members as a group came close together. By then, says Nell, she was happy, very happy, for the first time in her

life, to be a woman. Nell couldn't pull together with the
socialists and the feminists in those days. She knew you
couldn't have women's liberation without changing the
nature of power and you couldn't change the nature of
power without recognising women. Women didn't have
power and so Nell, from a socialist stand-point, made a big
shift to feminism. It was, of course, the conundrum of the
group. That, and the fact that it was such hard work. After
the launching of the movement in the Mansion House,
when there were twenty groups, all of whom had demands,
considerations, local problems, it became obvious that we
had bitten off more than we could chew. We didn't know
enough to manage the force we had created.

"And we didn't want to know," claims Nell. "We were
tired and the movement had confronted us with our own
personal dilemmas and that sort of thing takes a lot of
time and energy. I knew a woman there who was about to
marry a man because she loved him but didn't want
marriage, a woman who wanted to marry to go straight,
just to relax, a woman who was divorced, a woman who
was living with a dying man, a woman whose husband was
on his way out and loved somebody else, a woman who
loved her husband but couldn't cope with living with him
because he was a male chauvinist. And there was this
constant tension between socialism and feminism, which
was not clearly identified, plus there were the masses. We
were so happy with each other and then suddenly, we had
to cope with the masses, and it's hard fuckin' work."

Nell went on with the breakaway core which changed
the name from Irish Women's Liberation Movement to the
Women's Liberation Movement in Ireland on the grounds
that that was non-sectarian. It met in Fownes Street and
became known as the Fownes group. Nell says she sat
around with the rest while they discussed every problem in
the world except theirs, and split hairs all over the place.
The group attempted to deal with sexual politics: to
understand what was going on between themselves and
men. And as for the masses, the women everywhere who
had tuned into us, Nell says: "We turned them on, tuned

them in, Jesus they thought they had problems. Didn't we?" Nell may have been a bit more tired of fighting than the rest of us by the time the Irish Women's Liberation group broke up. She'd been up to the hilt in the Civil Rights struggle at a time when she wouldn't have realised that contraception was a civil right, that a person's sexual preference is a civil right and that the slogan "one man, one vote" is sexist.

I hadn't seen Nell for ages when I bumped into her one day coming down Grafton Street and asked her what she'd been doing? "Nothin' much, unless you count crawling on my belly dodgin' bullets", she replied, delighted by the expression on my face, "you been doing anything exciting?" Nell had gone for the Internment March on 30 January 1972, and became part of Bloody Sunday. It started, she recalls, with the soldiers shooting an old man and a teen-ager. It was about 4 o'clock and "these two wee boys arrived around the flats, one of them with red hair, real macho like John Wayne and I said 'for fuck sake, go away on home.' And they went home. And I was standing at the gate to the high flats in the courtyard and there was a wee barricade and suddenly soldiers came sweeping through and there were shots. It could have been rubber bullets, it could have been guns and these four wee fellows were in front of me. I saw them fall and said to Patsy Murphy 'we got to get out of here, it's getting dangerous'." They ran to a woman's door with Nell yelling "Missus, missus, let us in." She did. "Then these two fellows arrived and said to me 'let us in' and just as he said it soldiers arrived at the entrance to the courtyard and shots rang out and the fellow fell in front of me. I closed the door because I knew he had been shot and I looked out the window. His name was Nash, I discovered later, and he looked up and said: 'help me' and I said to Patsy, 'Christ, if you open that door you'll be killed' and he was lying there shouting help and there was another fellow there. I knew they were both dying but there was no way I was going out because I would have been killed. And I bent down and suddenly there were all these bullets and I heard

219

the window next door breaking. Soldiers firing recklessly. We stayed in the house for about ten minutes and then I was curious and I looked out and the guy was dying and then this nurse with a Red Cross uniform came into the courtyard and we were looking out and she went to touch one of the guys, not the one at the door or on the foot-path, but another guy in the middle of the courtyard and the soldiers started shooting at her and she danced around the bullets. Up against a wall was Dennis Bradley, the priest, and there was about twenty or thirty more rounded up against the wall with their hands up being searched and I could see them putting the four wee fellows off the barricade into a jeep. Across the courtyard I could see this doctor called Ray McClean gesticulating at the troops and not being shot at, and I knew it was all over and came out. McClean became mayor of Derry. The fellow at the door was dead and we left him. Barney McFadden was lying there and somebody was doing something with a matchbox which I later discovered was his eyelid being put in a matchbox. That fellow had died in front of me and I didn't open the door. I couldn't. We went home."

All the reporters went to Nell's house and Bernadette Devlin was on the 'phone saying: "I'm Bernadette Devlin, the MP." They told her who was dead and she kept writing names through the day. Later, a young girl, one of the McDaids from down the road, came to the house asking if anyone had seen "our Hugh?" Nell hadn't seen him, but her sister Carmel had been lying with him in the barricade and then got away without him.

'The sister came in again at about half-six and said 'he's dead, my brother, what am I going to do?' And she came into the house screaming. I can't remember whether we told her he was dead or not or let her go to the hospital or back to her mother's house. We sent out for a Chinese supper. I refused to believe it was all happening."

One of the Derry stories Nell used to tell was about fourteen-year-old Oxo. Oxo had a friend called Mad Dog because of his behaviour, who eventually got a stiff jail sentence. Meanwhile Oxo got married, had children, separated from his wife, was on the dole and looked the worst of it. The fact that his beautiful teeth went bad affronted Nell, especially when she met Mad Dog released from prison, calm, educated from the books he had read there and with excellent teeth. She met him again at the funeral of Patsy O'Hara (the hunger striker) and he said to her: "The town looks very dirty ..." "Why wouldn't it?" asked Nell, "after you tryin' to wreck it before you went into prison?" Nell ponders over who has come off best, Mad Dog with his prison sentence or Oxo with his teeth rotted.

Oxo got his name because instead of tea, where the kids in Derry played the juke box and hung out, he bought Oxo because "it feeds" he told Nell. She referred to him as "a child of our times, no mother's son living in a no man's land called Free Derry. Mothers were all we had and he didn't have one."

Nell sat talking to him for an hour when she first met him. The other boys jeered Oxo saying "you've got a girl" and Oxo kissed Nell. She kissed him back, nearly twice his age, and adopted him, or rather let her mother adopt him. He used to come home to their house every day to eat and when he threw stones, Nell asked him not to go too far forward or to wear a mask.

Oxo got married at eighteen and Nell was furious at the Credit Union for giving him £400. The loan started him off on a traditional way of living, but it maddened Nell thinking of him marrying so young and spending all the money on a wedding. One of Nell's sisters got him a job as a gravedigger in the cemetery, sometimes planting the roses, and he'd work at casual labour. Now he works in a community set-up in the parish and teaches football to girls, one of whom is Nell's niece.

Nell left the *Irish Times* because she felt her column, "In The Eyes of the Law" had come to an end. Partly, she was beginning to get irritated with these people appearing in court time after time and not changing their lives. Besides, she wanted to do more work. She was fed up. She felt she had a salary and was turning out mechanical shit.

She didn't want to be part of that any more and she wanted to write a novel about Derry. At that stage she could do her court column in half an hour. She'd stay in bed until two, go down to the court for ten minutes, write the thing in twenty minutes and be finished by five. "We were sent off like work-horses to record trivia and recorded it faithfully. I was worried that I'd become part of the bourgeois capitalist set up. I had been living with a woman who kept saying she was outside the system. I realise now she was outside the system because she couldn't get in. She'd beat me over the head all the time saying I was a capitalist pig. I worked less and less, with less and less enthusiasm, and the more I became like her the less she respected me." Then Nell met a woman who liked her career, liked to work, wanted to earn her own way and was prepared to support Nell for a while until Nell got on her feet as a writer. They went to live in Cork, delighted to get out of Dublin and leave that "silly, empty life, work until six, drink until ten, stagger home senseless into your bed. Holy Fuck."

Now Nell began to learn about making a home, the joy of cooking food, keeping the place clean and sitting at peace, not ego-tripping. She learned how the other half lives and it was not in confrontation. And then she returned to Dublin, with her novel begun. Her flat Derry voice saying hilarious, outrageous, true things began to be heard again on RTE's "Women Today" programme.

She had never supported the Provos; but suddenly women were involved, women, like men, were on the blanket in Armagh Jail and it was inevitable that she'd be involved. She called their plight a feminist issue and did battle with those of us who said it wasn't. She hadn't been too shocked by the blanket protest, because she didn't believe men were that concerned about cleanliness anyway. When did they clean lavatories? Besides that, her love of prisoners made her feel that it was wrong for them to look for special status, political status. She didn't believe in criminals. She believed that it wasn't a prisoner's fault he was in jail. But she was jolted when women joined the dirty protest. "I knew, wet liberal though I was, that these women were in this, not because they were anti-social or came from broken homes, but because of a war, and when a *woman* makes the total sacrifice, smearing shit on the walls, when there is menstrual blood involved, you have to look and say 'what's going on?' It was a lie to say that war is no part of feminism. People like Anne Speed and others kept saying: we have to be involved in the North. There was a war going on and what could we do? So I stepped in on the grounds that there were women suffering. I'd feel my way forward because I felt it was wrong that they were driven to that. That's how I got involved. Just because I'm a woman."

Marriage, believes Nell, is as traditional as nationalism, so if some women get married why shouldn't some women join the Provos? People join the Provos, she says, because they know there is a presence in Ireland and it must be ended. Those women were allowed to take up arms within the Provos the way women in the women's movement were allowed to operate outside the traditional women's rôle. Some people blame them for operating outside the traditional women's rôle; we drove them to it, says Nell, we expected them to do it. "I think people have a right to take up arms against an oppressor; in the occupied territory of Northern Ireland you are fighting to break out of British Imperialism."

Eventually, it occurred to Nell that she had been trying to be a husband to her mother, or rather give her the sort of recognition that she feels women do not get in marriage. Nell's father would open his pay packet every Friday night, as Nell remembers: "tore it open, big ceremony and gave her so much and he kept so much for himself, we never knew how much he was keeping. But we knew we were safe, that my father always paid his bills, we were never left in want in as much as it was within his control." That's what bugged her. It was totally within his control and her father was unaware that this was wrong. She recalls that after an argument on a Friday night, it would take an extra ten minutes to open the pay packet and the breadman would knock at the door and say, "Lily, I want to be paid" and she'd look as if to say, "I hope the row is over, because if I ask him for the money he might hold back." "Now my father wasn't to blame for that. He was brought up to think that the man provided. He held that power."

Nell always wanted to provide her mother with economic independence, to let her have enough money, to pay her for running a house, something which Nell has always thought beyond payment. No one I know appreciates more being given homely comforts and a meal put in front of her than Nell. She was perfectly aware of the service her mother gave her, of the services all mothers give, and this became even more obvious to her when she started trying to live by herself. "To be the cause of all that love spinning around you," Nell once mused, "always the place the rest of us went back to. Let alone produce food, cook you a meal, clean up the house ..."

Nell's mother didn't marry until she was twenty-eight because she had to rear her brother and sister. She brought her husband out of his rigidity; he had come from a very strict family. What Nell realises now is how good her father was to her mother, and she feels she would have been better to complement the deficiencies of her father than to try to replace him. But that was his problem, says Nell, in an effort to harden. "It's up to men to have their own liberation, and there's no way I'll take the blame, if they refuse to liberate themselves. I have tried to liberate myself and other women."

For herself, Nell sees her liberation in being a writer, in not having to do "awful, draining, draggy journalism. To do what I know to be right without hurting other people, to have love relationships without hurting anybody." She believes that we campaign for liberation in a society that has not yet grasped the point of liberation. What fascinates her is the way in which attempts to knit the running stitches of women's lives back into traditional garments has resulted in a dramatic call for the casting off of such garments. Ireland is still not ready for the cultural shock of divorce in a country which has cleaved to the idea of eternal marriage, nor for the effects of free and legal contraception and changing sexual behaviour patterns, nor for the effects of equal pay on Irish family life.

In her column "Equality" in the *Irish Times* in 1975, in a commentary on the Women's Year, Nell said: "It should be the function of feminism to see the connection between these disparate demands and to understand the nature of the radical change which will flow from them. The removal of women's oppression must obviously lead to a change in the economic base of society. This is most dramatically seen in the maintenance courts — you cannot equitably divide the labourer's wage between the deserted wife and her six children and the defecting husband. Several questions arise from that simple fact. Can a male breadwinner keep a family? Can a deserted mother keep a family on half the male breadwinner's wages? Should motherhood, an essential job, be unpaid? If motherhood is to be a paid job, will it be paid on the scale of the editorship of the *Irish Times* or that of the agricultural worker? Do socialists, who pose these questions, advocate pay for the home-maker, meaning woman or man, or are they still thinking in terms of wife and mother? And if so, how many male socialists are fighting for the right to get back in the home?" Until these questions are posed, Nell believes we will be left with a mere concept of equality. "Middle-class women might one day be economically equal to middle-class men. Working-class women might one day be economically equal to working-class men. Between the classes and the sexes there will still be divisions. And there'll be no liberations at all."

12
THE SPLIT

The local groups set up before the Contraceptive Train varied in their awareness of feminism and in their activities. We had cracked the surface of consciousness and were surprised by much of what emerged.

There were the same old divisions of class, left versus right, so there was from the beginning a difference of opinion as to what our six demands should be. Some were totally dependent on having the Founder's Group, as we were now called, at meetings. But other groups were as strong as ever we had been. Represented by Hilary Orpen, a presenter in Telefís Éireann, the Sutton group produced a magazine almost immediately. They announced their objectives: "1. To concentrate on an initial campaign to implement the Constitution of this State with regard to women. 2. To encourage women to take action on specific issues affecting them by whatever means seem appropriate at the time and to support such action. 3. To see as a long term objective the function of making all women aware of their exploitation in all areas of life, including those not covered in the Constitution (commercial exploitation through manipulation, civil rights not recognised in this State, such as divorce, etc.)." They had set themselves up in the same way as the original group without elected officers and with the minutes being taken by the member in whose house the meeting was held.

The first activity in which they were involved was a lobby outside Leinster House, concerning Senator Mary

Robinson's Contraceptive Bill. One of their members was asked by a TD to "cool the pressure". The answer was an emphatic "No".

We had been refused admission to the Dáil on that occasion and Hilary Orpen had climbed through the window of the men's toilet in the basement with Máirín de Burca and Fionnuala O'Connor. Máirín later remarked that it was an "escape" to get them away from the "excruciating" sound of Mary Kenny singing "We Shall Not Conceive" to the air of "We Shall Overcome". However, I remember that when the three were escorted out we were all determinedly singing.

The Eurovision Song Contest was picketed. Prior to Ireland's entry to the EEC, it was considered important that we should inform the Europeans of Ireland's backwardness in relation to contraception. Leaflets handed to foreign personalities pointed to the fact that contraception in any form was illegal in Ireland. One wonders if some of those show biz people mightn't have feared there'd be gardai under their hotel beds. Ireland, explained the leaflet, as a member of the United Nations, was not bound by this organisation's Universal Declaration of Human Rights (Article 54). The Sutton group took it into their own hands to picket the housing of three priests in separate houses when families were left unhoused. There were pickets outside the GPO over the paying of Children's Allowances. The forms stipulated that the husband must nominate his wife before she was eligible to sign for her Children's Allowance.

The Clonskeagh group got steam up over the sexist advertisements in their area, with stickers reading "this is insulting to women". The founder group was anxious to reach agreement on the six demands of the movement. There was still the old tension around "one family, one home". It was impossible to get enough time to travel around to all the group meetings and Mary Anderson, Fionnuala O'Connor and Marie McMahon seemed to do more than their share, all being freer to do so. A few of us took a lorry up to Ballymun one Saturday afternoon and I remember it as the beginning of a hectic though short career on lorry platforms with Kevin Clear campaigning against the EEC. The Ballymun gig was memorable because I was supposed to pick up the microphone and hail the women from the high-rise flats doing their weekly shop: "Women of Ballymun," I called and was ignored, again and again. "Louder," said Nell McCafferty, "you're not at a tea-party."

"Women of Ballymun," I began again, suddenly becoming conscious of my own middle-class voice. I handed the thing to Nell and she immediately gathered a crowd.

"Who sent for ye?" asked a Ballymun woman with three children under four years, "Who's doing your shoppin' while yez are talkin' at us?" It wasn't a question that was ever answered, but the Ballymun group, represented by Patsy Kelly of Sean McDermott Tower, became one of the more active groups. Their protest against the fact that they had to walk a mile to the nearest post-office to pick up their husbands' Children's Allowance got national media coverage.

Quite a few local groups would not accept the "one house, one family" demand or take part in events such as the May Day March. And now, there were objections to men being excluded from meetings. Not strangely, it was the least confident groups who wanted men present, but this issue arose in the founder group too.

In August of that year, about three hundred members of the Irish Women's Liberation Movement protested outside Leinster House against the Forcible Entry Bill which, after a guillotined debate, was being forced through the Dáil that night. This issue always split us in two. Now, I believe it was not, strictly speaking, a feminist issue, but then as it was a Bill opposing squatters it seemed part of an overall struggle against the forces which oppressed women. Women were the primary victims of lack of housing, the weight falling mainly on their shoulders, as was the case with those families housed at Griffith Barracks. The state had dealt with these families for non-payment of rent by putting them into dormitory accommodation. In retrospect,

I see the Bill as having been a big distraction, creating splits and confusion, but if a woman's place was in the home and she didn't have a home, then surely?

We might have sorted that out if there hadn't been quite so many very strong women, uncontrolled by any structure. Élitism was charged, although I think the word was used to describe people within the founder group who had naturally developed bonds and closeness which later arrivals could not penetrate quickly. Impatience was an important factor. There was such an urgency in the atmosphere, such pent-up energy. The groups were making statements that were taken as representative of the entire movement. The meetings over Gaj's had become impossible because of the numbers of delegates who wished to attend and the fact that we could never get on with our own business. It was expected of us that we go over issues with each group after we had been over that ground time and time again ourselves. It was also vital if the groups were to merge and unite that the founder group should have a chance of discussing the development of the local groups, but we couldn't do it while they insisted on being there.

By now, some of us would have given anything for a bit of reliable structure, to settle for a proven way of getting things done for a while. It was agreed that we organise to bring about a more co-ordinated programme and philosophy representing the Movement as a whole. A document was drawn up, suggesting that the founders' group should remain thus, with a membership of about twenty. Other groups should be encouraged to form in whatever locale women found themselves, with four or five members sufficient to start a group. Any member of the founders' group who wished to start a new group could, of course, do so; new members could be recruited to the maximum number agreed on as workable.

Bureaucracy in administration was to be avoided at all costs. A Steering Committee of four or five would be elected to attend to managerial duties. Decisions on active tactics were to be taken by each group independently, co-ordinated and organised by voluntary effort. No member could be compelled to participate in any specific action; no member ever had been. The movement should operate on a "popular democracy" basis in that it would have no spokeswomen or conventional leaders. This would be compatible with our aim of involving all women to take an active part in the campaign and not merely to exercise a vote and wait passively for the elected representatives to take charge. Any member could give statements, quotes, etc. as long as she made it clear that she spoke as an individual. The chairwoman's position would be taken in rotation. All would be entitled to promulgate the agreed objectives included in the charter at any and every opportunity. The objectives were as published by the Sutton group. However, individual groups and individual members should be free to offer support and encouragement where and when needed and without seeking the express consent of others in the movement. This, it was stressed, was in line with the ideal of the Movement as a broad based campaign, one that agreed to allow differences within its ranks on tactics or priorities.

To some, it looked like the same old chaotic structure with everybody doing their own thing. To others it looked like the founder group taking over, giving the orders. The honeymoon was over.

Euphoria was replaced by weariness and in-fighting. People were missing meetings. I was amazed to see "Women's Lib Takes A Body Blow" written across the front page of the paper lying on a pile at the bus stop one night. Nuala Fennell, a founder member of the IWLM had claimed bitterly that "Women's Lib has not only lost her virginity but has turned into a particularly nasty harlot" and added that she was joining the "mass" of members now resigning in disgust. Realising that the idea of the movement having taken a body blow was a sub-editor's fantasy, I was nonetheless amazed at the force with which Nuala attacked us, more amazed that anyone thought herself important enough to write a letter to the national papers about her resignation from the group. It was the first glimpse of Nuala, the politician, even though we didn't realise it then:

> As one of the founder members of the Irish Women's Liberation Movement, who is now resigning, it comes as no surprise to me to hear of the mass resignations in nearly all the newly formed groups in all the twenty-five Dublin postal districts. For one thing, it proves that Irishwomen, for all the discriminations and deprivations they suffer, are not the blinkered female donkeys that the small policy-making central group of Women's Liberationists thought them to be.

She claimed that Women's Lib. was being used as a pseudo-respectable front by those anxious to achieve their own political ends, ranging from opposition to the Forcible Entry Bill to providing free sedatives for neurotic elephants. "At a recent seminar it was clearly stated that if any member, whatever her previous views, was not against the aforementioned bill, then she was not in Women's Lib ... and to this I can add authoritatively that if you are not anti-American, anti-clergy, anti-Government, anti-ICA, anti-police, anti-men, then, sisters, there is no place for you either."

The "anti-American" charge referred to those people active against the Vietnamese war. Anti-clergy and anti-Government hardly needed explaining in the context of feminism. Anti-police referred to those who were constantly confronting the police in those days of political demonstrations. What the anti-Irish Countrywomen's Association charge was about was hard to say.

> Perhaps this development was a foreseeable trend, the Women's Lib. group now in America being the radical trouble-making anti-Establishment group. It is the National Organization of Women (NOW) who are achieving reforms and concessions. At present I believe there is interest in such a group being formed in Dublin, who would hope to work on the national in-

equalities, concentrating on reform of the law and it might be the answer for those women who have been put out or off by Women's Lib.

Most of the original founder group truly and emphatically believed the frustrations and malcontent of the opting out that being a woman can mean, and were totally dedicated to group consciousness-raising and self-education while at the same time fighting a campaign to right the wrongs. For me, it would be funny if it weren't sad, being discriminated against by the group for being middle-class when they are all unquestionably that and trying hard not to show it.

My last meeting at which regional delegates attended, heard one sane voice (Mary Kenny's) exhort us not to lose our identity in disproportionately fighting the housing problem or community schools, these issues being, in fact, the bread and butter of other political groups — that it could be suicide for us. Her plea is too late, I'm afraid. Women's Lib. has not only lost her virginity, but has turned into a particularly nasty harlot, and in all fairness it is on this level she will be dealt with by the majority of Irish men and women.

As Nuala Fennell resigned on the grounds of Women's Lib. being involved in too many political activities, another well-known member, Hilary Boyle, who at almost seventy was a couple of decades older than anyone else in the group, resigned for the opposite reasons. She attacked Women's Lib because of our lack of interest in real problems like housing, squatting, Rachman rents. "I believe that helping people such as these is one hundred times more important than the eternal and non-ending talk of contraception," she wrote, "wherefore let it be known that I resign." Of course families should be limited, "but house all decently and family planning will follow as naturally as night follows day. I am sickened by single girls talking nothing but contraception, instead of getting on with the work that needs doing."

The letters summed up the main split in the movement, but the writers were clearly unaware of subconscious difficulties evolving from structure and expansion. There now followed a wrangle through the letters columns of the papers. Nell McCafferty said it was unfortunate that Nuala Fennell's absence from meetings should lead her to issue a statement saying exactly what Women's Lib had been saying for months. "No political philosophy, be it right, left or centre, has taken over Women's Lib. The aims of the movement are entirely intended to lead towards the new society and equality of life in which there would be true liberation for all people." Máirín Johnston, the group's PRO and most popular member, pointed out that the twenty-five groups had now risen to thirty-three. Further, that Nuala's three previous resignations had been withdrawn before we could accept. She defended the group's policies: "Supporting the aim of One Family, One House necessitates opposing the Forcible Entry and Occupation Bill. This was decided unanimously at a delegate meeting at which Nuala Fennell was present. She did not voice any objections. It was never intended that the IWLM would be a conservative movement. Of course we are radical — we are going to change society ...

"The question of whether men should be admitted is at present under discussion in all groups and no decision has yet been reached. We are not anti-man and the accusation is as tired as the accusation of subversion.

"As for her views on free sedatives for elephants, life in the human jungle is no joke; most of the available sedatives are unfortunately needed for women. We intend to change that situation. Those who disagree should pack their trunks."

Laura Conroy of the Sutton group saw Nuala's criticisms as being recommendations for the movement: "Of course we are anti-police, anti-government, anti-EEC and anti-the Prohibition and Forcible Entry Bill. If we can make a farce of the law by one contraceptive train to Belfast we will do the same to any other dictatorial measures the Government chooses to force upon us ... Nuala, you had better stick to

NOW, the ICA or any other women's guild that does not question your fundamental beliefs in your husband and the society that he and his colleagues have so glibly produced for us."

Furious letters continued to rage. Nuala claimed our allegations against her were wrong, she had attended a meeting on 12 June. Hilary Boyle charged that Laura Conroy's letter was a sign that Women's Lib did not stand for freedom but slavery to the addle-pated few, all solidly middle-class, who would be the first to object if they had itinerants at the bottom of their gardens or homes for the poorer working class erected next door to them.

That letter came to my mind years later when a travelling family parked themselves at the bottom of my garden. Our house was set well back from the road. I don't know where they had their caravan but every morning around eleven the mother and five children would appear beneath the seven foot wall, sheltered by trees, and proceed with their daily living. Every day I would give the family something, sweets, biscuits and a few bob. Always, the woman and myself exchanged blessings. It's true we grew no friendlier, but ...

One Monday I had put two chickens into a casserole in the oven. It was a lovely day and I took off for a walk. I brought some biscuits, but had no money. No matter. I wouldn't need any till the bank opened tomorrow. Down I went to my itinerant family, wincing at the sight of garbage strewn about the garden. I handed the biscuits round to the children and remarked on the beauty of the day to the mother. Had I e'er something towards feeding them? "I'm sorry, I haven't any money in the house today, but if I could help some other way?" She ignored that, starting to speak before I'd finished. Her voice went on and on, with that world-wide determination of beggars, about the childer and not a bit since last Friday and himself drinkin' hard again.

I'd never set eyes on himself. Now, I saw that the children had not fallen on the chocolate biscuits with anything like three days' hunger. The smallest one held up the biscuit for me to unwrap. I explained that I hadn't any money. Yes, I could get some, but not until to-morrow. I had groceries in the house, what did she need? But the voice drove on, using up the air between us. I stood there for ages, having what felt like a conversation with a computerised wall. Finally, I offered: "Look, when I come back you can bring the kids in and I'll cook some vegetables to go with the chicken. There's plenty for both families." The voice pressed on. I offered the chicken again, thinking at the back of my mind would I ask the man who owned the nearby supermarket to lend me some money. Suddenly, the computer seemed to blow a gasket, spluttering and roaring while the mother sprang up from where she had been slouched on a blanket on the grass and thrust her blazing face into mine: "Ya fuckin' cunt ..."

"The likes of you" was a phrase that stuck out, the *you* seeming a filthy thing held by a tongs at arm's length. When she got round to telling me what himself would do to me next time I came up the dark avenue, I simply ran from her. It was only on the walk back I remembered her terrible life, how natural was her resentment and distrust of my class. And how inventive had been her sexual fantasy for "himself" and me. I wished she'd move on, but she stayed and stayed. Every time I came home after dark, I'd ring to ask someone to come to the gate and meet me off the bus. Always, I thought of Hilary Boyle. "Sisterhood, me arse," as one of my friends would say. It reminds me of my artist brother Les when he was aged four and I told him there were fairies at the bottom of the garden, but to see them you had to believe in them. "And do they believe in us?" he asked.

Nuala Fennell, TD and Fine Gael spokeswoman on women's affairs has written that when her grandchildren ask her what she did in Women's Lib, she'll tell them she left and started all over again.

"With herself as boss," echo many of those who remember. Emerging from the nappy buckets, beginning a career as a free-lance journalist, Nuala seemed anxious to be in command. In appearance, there was a neat, no nonsense air about her, as if she were in uniform. She avoided emotion, frivolity, intimate conversation. She was terribly underestimated by the group, possibly because although she obviously had a drive to power, she lacked charisma.

The image of the driven woman came across worst on television. She had the courage and conviction to push herself in front of the TV cameras at every opportunity. "Nuala Fennell," TV researchers would say, "is her own worst enemy. She doesn't rant or shout like Kenny and the rest of you, but she looks so fierce. A dragon."

By then, in 1972, she had formed AIM (Action, Information, Motivation), the first pressure group spawned by the Irish Women's Liberation Movement, and people were loath to hear what Nuala had to say about the state of so many Irish marriages. Always, when she spoke about the agony of Irish marriage gone sour, she prefaced it by saying she was a happily married woman, married to the same man for years (as if it could be otherwise in Ireland), before launching into the plight of deserted wives.

AIM grew out of Nuala's local branch of the IWLM with Deirdre McDevitt and Bernadette Quinn and about a dozen others, including Nuala's husband Brian and some other men. It was reformist and traditionally-structured and Nuala had tight hold of the reins. The goal was a campaign of law reform in areas related to women and the family. It had always been Nuala's belief that one thing at a time would get things done for women, with each group concentrating on a specific aim. That was a recommendation of the National Commission on the Status of Women in 1973. By this system, Nuala Fennell had managed to do a great deal for the women of Ireland. In return, they have gone to the polls and given Nuala their votes.

Peter Prendergast advised that the task of AIM be undertaken gradually, tackled slowly, systematically. There were never more than eighteen in the group, and they got their first report out in twelve months. They accepted that to change public opinion and to avoid alienation it was wise to step carefully, to say "here's what's needed", to explain the human need. Prendergast advised that they plan for a five year span, at a time when groups were springing up all over the place and everybody wanted things done yesterday. Although Prendergast, who had founded the Consumer Association, was non-political in those days, he was Fine Gael National Party Secretary in 1981 and master-minded the election which brought Nuala into the Dáil.

AIM forced Irish people to admit that marriages broke down here, seemingly no less often than elsewhere. "Divorce Irish style" too often meant desertion by the breadwinner. Nuala's voice revealed that deserted Irish wives lived in poverty, shame and isolation, worse than invisible in a society that did not believe in their existence.

In retrospect, it seems obvious that Irish society would accept the distressed wife as a charitable cause. The important thing was that *marriage* was not being questioned. No one was being blamed except "the law". The deserted wife became an institution. She wasn't asked to fight. She would be rescued. Poor woman. After all, what could she do if himself abandoned her? Besides, what about the unfortunate children?

Nuala's empathy with the deserted wife had come from her own fierce sense of independence. As a young wife with small children, she was keenly aware of her vulnerability. Publicly, she never said that. She had an instinct for knowing how to leave conservative feathers unruffled. She sensed that Ireland saw reforms as sufficient liberation for women.

I was studying the Chinese values of *yin* and *yang,* masculine and female, in the early 'seventies and decided that Nuala was the most *yang* woman I knew, much more so than most of the so called "ravers" of the time. A dutiful and concerned mother, her masculine self was fighting to get out. She was like a little tomboy shaking off hair-ribbons, bound to prove herself as good as her brothers. She projected *yang* values, representing the culture in which she'd grown up. She favoured self-assertion over integration, the rational over the intuitive, the practical over the sentient, competition over co-operation and the task as concrete achievement above all else. I used to think that an example of her *yang* tendency was the fact that she had an office extension built on to her house when the rest of us still worked off our kitchen tables. She also acquired a personal hideaway in the country. Now, I realise she simply wasn't as badly conditioned against her own needs as most of us. Over time, Nuala going from strength to strength has become increasingly more fulfilled, at peace with herself as a woman, surely disproving the myth that achievement in a man's world destroys female values.

AIM fought for Family Maintenance Legislation, The Family Home Protection Act (so that a husband couldn't sell the roof over his wife's head without her agreement) and barring orders against violent husbands. It published reports on all that, and on legal separation in Ireland. It held seminars and campaigned successfully to have the Children's Allowance transferred from father to mother. (These funds were referred to as "mickey money" by Dublin's working class, saluting the organ from which they multiplied). The real work of AIM, the gruelling day-to-day work, apart from planning, lobbying, seminars and publications, was the support of deserted wives, answering their letters, talking to them, helping them to sort out their lives. This work had uncovered the horrendous problem of family violence, of beaten, tortured and raped wives and terrified children, of all kinds of hell within the home. It was a slow process, getting the facts of Irish marriage breakdown across to those who could help change things. In 1974, Nuala wrote *Irish Marriage, How Are You?*, a book which was not pretty reading.

She stepped into her hallway very late one night after a meeting to have Brian rush her in to the television. The BBC was showing "Scream Quietly Or The Neighbours Will Hear", which interviewed some women who had run away to London from Irish husbands. At the time, Nuala had been struggling with the problem of a woman with six children living in a well-to-do neighbouring suburb. The woman was hospitalised and could not go home. She knew other women driven out of their homes by violence, with nowhere to go. After the BBC show, she wrote a letter to the *Irish Times,* metaphorically laying the foundations for the first Irish Women's Aid Committee. I was working as a researcher on the "Late Late" when Nuala asked Erin Pizzey of London's Women's Aid to come and tell the Irish people about family violence. Rolf Harris, the Australian entertainer on the show that night, broke down in tears, moved by the stories of young Irish women on the panel.

At about the same time as she set up Women's Aid, AIM opened an advice centre for women, the house being offered to them by a property developer who had watched Erin Pizzey. Another arm of AIM was ADAPT, a support group for single parents where they could learn to cope with the day-to-day personal and emotional problems of living in Ireland's limbo of broken marriages.

Women's Aid proved to be a next to impossible task for Nuala. The work was intense and unending and any day could as easily find her with her arm down a lavatory, unplugging the plumbing, as making a case to a politician or supporting a woman in court. With Fr. Chris Crowley, Brian tried to run a rehabilitation course for violent husbands. It did not work. The husbands believed that their wives were their property with which they could do as they pleased. The effort drained Brian's health. Nuala departed from Women's Aid under some controversy. She believed the place should be run with control, house rules. The committee disagreed. It was getting too much to cope with a houseful of helpless broken mothers and disturbed children who seemed intent on pulling the place apart.

Anyone who has ever visited the Dublin centre for battered wives is appalled to realise how bad must be the places from which these families fled, if they are relieved to be allowed to live in this "refuge". Women's Aid has always suffered from insufficient funds. Its struggle for existence as a voluntary group, getting a bit of money from the Health Board and the EEC, proves that the survival of the fittest is all that counts, even in a country which lauds the family in its Constitution. Why is it that a family under a physical, emotional, and economic attack should have no refuge provided by a Christian state? Why are the good family people of Ireland not marching the streets in protest against such an outrage? There is an answer but it is difficult to accept.

Nuala Fennell was the daughter of a garda sergeant named Patrick Campbell. When she talks about her late father, I can see him there in herself: "He was distant [although she is not that], disciplined, and feared a little bit. He expected to be obeyed and we were a bit in awe of him. He was an extraordinarily honest man with a fierce sense of right and justice. He had a sense of pure morality and was a religious man. By the time I was doing anything in public, he was aware, for instance, that he had tried to dissuade me from going away to Canada with Brian when I was twenty. He knew he couldn't tell me what to do. He didn't like the idea of me standing for politics, thought it a cheek. I really only got to know him in the last ten years of his life. He was a fine man."

Nuala's mother, Elizabeth Gallogly, "is absolutely traditional on the exterior, but I suspect underneath a woman's libber who would not let herself be seen as such. She believes that men have to be looked after. We fought it out between us. She thought when I first appeared in public that I was making a show of myself." A middle-class Dubliner, Elizabeth had been a super secretary with a hectic social life and more than one suitable beau. For a long time, says Nuala, her mother hoped she could slap her rebel daughter down and get her into line, and it took a while for her to realise that she couldn't. "She never got over my kicking a nun in the Convent of Mercy when I was three," says Nuala affectionately.

The Campbells lived in the married quarters of Garda barracks in Kells, Meath and Portlaoise before coming to Dublin when Nuala was twelve. She attended the Dominican Convent in Eccles Street, and her father bought a grocery shop in Blackrock. She went to commercial college and worked as a receptionist, typist and general Girl Friday for a tea importers' company on Bachelor's Walk. She earned

£2.10s.0d. a week, wore a navy overall, and resented it. She hated the sense of being caught in the herd. She was quite sure she would not get married. Did not *want* to get married. She was sorting a file one day when the manager said "now, Miss Campbell, you are eligible for a pension scheme ..." She was shocked at the idea that she could possibly still be there when she was old enough to draw a pension.

The first time Nuala met Brian at the Templeogue Tennis Club Saturday night dance, she told him she was never getting married. It was a ladies' choice. He was immediately fascinated. She claims that Brian just persistently stalked her: "I was not the sort of person to fall madly or instantly in love." Eventually, they went off to Canada, engaged. There in 1958, Nuala was impressed by women she met who had their own incomes and consequent freedom. Still, she wanted to come home. They came back and got jobs and eventually they married. With three children — Garrett (who now intends to be a politician), Jacqueline (who is at university) and Mandy — Nuala was not quite the typical pre-woman's movement archetype of the 'sixties. She had wanted children, but she found housewifery and motherhood a tyranny. Brian, she says now, understood better than she did herself: "I was awful for some time, irritable, weepy, half here, half somewhere else. I wanted to do something else with my life and yet I loved my family ..."

In 1969, Nuala's ambition was to become a journalist. She was looking out of her sitting room on a summer's day when she saw a scene so crazy, it drove her to put it on paper. There was an advertising firm with actors and a film crew, working on a soup ad. They'd turned the location into a freezing winter's day, the better to have the hot soup appreciated by the TV family. Seán McCann of the *Evening Press* published the piece Nuala wrote and she was on her way.

In the mid-seventies people had begun to talk about Nuala as "a natural for politics". She pooh-poohed the idea until 1977 when it became obvious that the political parties were not about to fall over themselves in the attempt to put forward women candidates. There was much anger among women when obvious party choices such as Monica Barnes of Fine Gael, then on the executive of The Council for The Status of Women, were ignored for election nominations. Fired with desperation and annoyance, Nuala decided she'd run herself, as an Independent. It was an even harder choice than it looked on the face of things at the time. Brian was not well. However, no women had been selected to run in South County Dublin, and "how were we ever supposed to find out how they would do?" asked Nuala.

If they noticed at all, politicians were amused. Feminists were worried that her political failure would set back the women's cause. But she wasn't asking for anyone's permission. On 30 May, 1977, Nuala changed the beds, vacuumed the house and began her campaign for the General Election, a campaign which was designed as much to take the myth out of elections for women as to get Nuala into power. She produced a scripted manifesto, a photograph and the new logo "Why Not a Woman?" put out by the Women's Political Association, and took herself off to a printers for 35,000 simple black-and-white handouts. They had a calculated appeal to voters, and meeting Nuala at the time I realised that she knew little more than any other voter about General Elections. Government Information couldn't tell her what to do next, but she figured she needed envelopes, Voters' Registers, the Election Act and a map. She made contact with Liam Byrne, the Deputy Returning Officer for South County Dublin. She registered with the Sheriff, using her own £100. People started to phone, to send money, offer help, to say she was crazy. One woman sent £500. Nuala started thinking "Jesus, what have I done?" Her father didn't talk to her for the entire campaign. He resented her running against Liam Cosgrave, previous leader of Fine Gael.

"Men," said Nuala, "make an awful fuss about things like politics, and they are supported by office staff, wives, a back-up fabric that maintains the myth. I had to look after my family at the same time. D'you remember the panic when Communion shoes had to be bought ..."

I do indeed. I was excited by Nuala's spunk and offered my help. It was only then I got to know Nuala properly, rather than by impression. She was energetic, cheerful and generous, always ready to laugh and yet totally identified with the problems of women. I trudged around her constituency, always lost in a maze of houses, forever searching for the first house in a row so I could start. Like Nuala, I was amazed at the helplessness of individuals, of their inability to find out about things, to know what they were entitled to, to understand how much or how little power politicians have. We were also moved by how much responsibility women took in their families. They worried about every member, themselves last.

As the campaign got under way, Brian, who had been unwell, seemed to gather strength so that he became a gentle driving support. But what a politician really needs is a wife. The children still had to eat, people were coming and going to the house — and my feet were killing me. I remember the occasion that decided me to give up canvassing and take over cooking for Nuala. A door was opened by a flustered woman who looked at the leaflets in my hand: "Oh God, not now!" and she ran back into her house shouting over her shoulder: "ah come in, then." As I arrived in her kitchen she was looking at two sides of a sponge sandwich on the kitchen table. Shrunken: too little flour. It was her son's birthday cake. "Look," I said, "if you listen to me while I work I'll throw another one in the oven for you!" She listened as I threw and the sponge came out a dream. We had a cup of tea while it was baking and as I was leaving she said: "I'll give my number one to Nuala Fennell, but I'm glad you didn't ask me to give it to a mad women's libber like that June Levine. I couldn't do that."

And so I cooked my way through the rest of the election, never questioning my rightful share in the celebrations when Nuala did so well. Nuala got 3,850 votes. We didn't realise how well she was doing until a man in the counting centre said: "you've done so well with first preferences ..." Some of the men around looked as if they'd had their lollipops snatched and might cry. Over a pizza with the Fennell family that evening, Nuala reflected: "It's unbelievable what we've done in three weeks. Who was it said women are a sleeping giant? Do you know women came from the other side of the city to canvass? Women got me those votes."

Nuala wasn't in the Dáil this time, but she'd exploded the myth. Women were released into politics. For now, it was back to deserted wives, journalism with a new crusading column in the *Evening Herald,* and the publication of *Can You Stay Married?* co-authored with Bernadette Quinn and Deirdre McDevitt.

Fine Gael asked her to contest the European Election two years later, and she came in second. In 1981 she got a Fine Gael seat in Dáil Éireann. She had been encouraged by Garret FitzGerald, who was politically courting females at the time, whether as successful candidates or voters. She was not warmly welcomed in her local branch of Fine Gael. Seeking nomination was a harder battle than the general election. "Most of them wouldn't even say hello to me or exchange pleasantries, and I had to go up to people and say 'I'm Nuala Fennell'." When I 'phoned her home one night, Brian told me that Nuala was off in her grovelling boots. The "grovelling" didn't pay off. She was not nominated and all hell broke loose. Typically Nuala, she declared the foolishness and prejudice of this. Opponents, especially in the guise of political writers, were at pains to point out that she had no right to protest, that there were others more deserving of nomination who were silent. Others perhaps, but not others with her record of votes, nor running on a women's ticket. Garret FitzGerald as party leader, imposed Nuala as his own personal choice of candidate in the area.

The day Nuala Fennell TD took her seat in the Dáil was the second greatest day in her life, she told me, the first being the day she gave birth to her eldest child, Jacqueline. The morning before the Dáil opened, she was mobbed by women in Bewley's cafe. On the day, there were women everywhere, pleading to be let into the House, delighted, elated, Nell McCafferty beside herself with joy explaining desperately: "but I have to get in to see Nuala Fennell." For Nuala it was not quite as awesome as she had expected it to be. There was a moment though, a moment in which she felt as if some man would come along and claim her place. And all around were the dark blue business suits. It was lovely, said Nuala, to see the eleven women out of 166 people in the Dáil, all dressed up. She wore a mint green dress and jacket. "Slimming and fresh" was how she described this concession to fashion.

Brian wasn't there, because there was only one guest ticket and Nuala brought her mother. "It seemed so important to bring her," said Nuala, "down through the years she had put so much into supporting politics, been so behind my father's interest in Fine Gael, and with my father recently dead ..." Mrs. Campbell, who had been so uncomfortable with Nuala's political ambitions, mounted the steps to Leinster House alongside her daughter and started to weep. Nuala dried her up fast: "If there is going to be tears I'll take you home. No crying. This isn't a day for tears."

In her maiden speech in the Dáil Nuala Fennell expressed, for the first time ever there, a concise litany of the concerns of Irishwomen.

"We do not have a comprehensive public health nursing service, we do not have a comprehensive family planning service and our preventative and educational medical schemes leave much to be desired." As an example she gave the fact that the important breast cancer screening technique of mammography, available in other countries, was virtually unavailable in Ireland where there is an annual death rate of 500 women from this disease.

She spoke of our lack of play-schools in a country with the largest population of small children in Europe and the fact that we cannot finance a meaningful retraining programme for women in mid-life, and emphasised the need for maternity hospitals where women, not just the privileged few, could give birth with dignity. She declared the neglected list of women's needs as endless, and then went on to tell the deputies: "Hands off the housewives' allowance: you do not speak for Irish women. Wives and mothers of this state came out with their prams and toddlers on a wet day and put their approval of our proposed allowance on record. Do not treat them as nitwits, whose democratic choice is of so little value that it can be overruled in this House."

As she spoke, not even she could have guessed that women would not come forward to apply for the £9.60 a week due to them if they were married to tax-paying husbands. The application date was extended, but at the end of December 1981, only 16,000 of 35,000 eligible Irishwomen applied. The Coalition's Government fell over the Budget seven months later, and with that ceased any mention of an allowance for stay-at-home wives.

Nuala's colleague, Senator Gemma Hussey, was Fine Gael spokeswoman on Women's Affairs, while young Mary Flaherty got the junior Social Welfare Ministry on Poverty and the Family. It looked as if Nuala herself was being under-estimated in the Coalition team. In 1982, back in Opposition, she wrote in an article in the *Irish Press* that the Dáil was not interested in legislating for women's issues, that women could achieve more outside the Dáil than in it. On the same day that the article appeared, Garret FitzGerald pronounced Nuala front bench opposition spokeswoman on women's affairs.

Somewhere, I have a Christmas card with an old world painting of the Holy Family, and inside: "from Brian and Nuala Fennell, TD." I smiled when I saw the "TD", but then, she meant me to.

13
DAUGHTERS

Fear and cynicism were the main enemies of the new women's movement. The fear was understandable, often shared by feminists themselves. Just because we were committed to change didn't stop us finding it personally frightening. Cynicism was worse. The most damaging kind came from women who knew the score. These were the women who knew very well that the game of playing at femininity had paid off for them in material terms. They knew how they got what they wanted. For the most part, they kept quiet, at least in public, but they were always there fuelling the anger and ridicule directed at feminists, expressing horror at the blue jeans and scrubbed faces of the movement. This last was a lousy trick, based on propaganda. There were jeans around, yes, but alas, most of us still got our hair done and wore make-up. Come to think of it, even people who did not normally wear make-up were made up in the TV studios before being allowed face the public, so what were people talking about? When else did they see or meet us?

"I'm cetainly not one of those libbers" was a remark, I noticed, usually accompanied by an ingratiating glance at the man present. We were called man-haters. Personally, indifference was more like it. I certainly couldn't have summoned up that much passion, willy-nilly, against all men. These cynical women were the real man-haters, it seemed to me. Still are. They didn't trust the human potential in any man, couldn't imagine that a man could change, might want to put an end to the injustice of the sex rôles even if it caused him inconvenience. So they backed off thinking about women's liberation because of a gut fear that such questioning would inevitably affect the way they felt about men, and hence affect their marriages.

Pretence was the barrier between them and the step to awareness which they feared would do them down. To them, a husband seen in a clear light was a fearful thought. Man-hating? Some women could teach feminists the real quality of hate, disrespect.

I had it explained to me by a thirty-year-old married woman: "OK, women can't afford to be nearly as romantic as men, but just the same, Western marriage is based on romantic concepts which every woman learns at her mother's knee — her father's knee, too for that matter — and must not be subject to too close examination. Honesty can ruin a marriage."

Bred in Co. Sligo, of well-heeled stock, she had previously expressed horror at the "marriage arrangements" of her parents, at the deadening transactions within their relationship. And yet she said: "I know Mike is a male chauvinist. I'm not going to let on I know. Not seriously. I'm going to work around it, and get what I want ..." Now, ten years on, the sad thing is that she didn't take the trouble to figure out what it was she wanted, for what she's got is something all too similar to her mother's marriage. Personally, I would have thought it a relatively simple matter to raise Mike's consciousness. He's a kind, logical man. But then I wasn't locked with him in the game of marriage.

My friend admits that something went wrong with their marriage relationship, but it's "reasonable" enough. Now, she says, if it was to do over again, she'd take the risk involved in changing her status in that marriage. She'd come clean, reveal her true sexual identity, her personal ambitions, her real strengths, her manipulative streak. Instead she got control of the strings so that now there they are, nice people, mainly puppets. My friend was seduced by comfort, crippled by her own lack of trust in the one she chose from that hateful species, men. I suppose it's hard to blame her. There were no rôle models of a different sort of marriage in those days. It takes a lot of courage to be a guinea-pig, break new ground in marriage. And yet isn't a relationship always new ground, hallowed ground? There seemed to her, then, to be no way of being seen to take control of one's life without threatening the relationship. I tried to help her. Her eyes reminded me that I was divorced.

On another level, women worried that they were being asked to be too strong for their own good. Were they being forced out into the work market? Who, again, could blame them for this? The jobs most women had left in the 'sixties and 'seventies were usually boring, repetitive, poorly paid, meant to be a stop-gap until they "succeeded" in getting a husband. Even if they were to go back to such jobs or somehow get better ones, they knew very well that because of the Irish tax system which discriminated against married women, adding the wife's money to the husband's and thereby taxing "his" total income, there would be little of their money left. The husband entered his wife's tax on his form; she had no right to know what he earned. Besides, who'd mind the children?

Banners in America in those early days blazoned "Starve A Rat Today" and "End Human Sacrifice, Don't Get Married". In London's subway was scrawled "Don't Be A Slave, Earn Your Own Bread". However, surveys in Germany, Britain, France and America at the time were showing that women with small children were not fleeing their homes. They were choosing to stay with them or take part-time jobs. Always rare, in fact, is the mother who does not *feel* child-rearing to be a vital social occupation, even if she knows it need not require twenty-four hours of her individual attention each day.

In 1970, it could be seen that the pattern of work was changing in the Western world. Yet few believed this. Mary Maher was considered radical by some and mad by others when she pointed out that the world of work would have utterly changed by the time our infant daughters of 1970 were grown. Family life would change as a result. Automation, said Mary, would make millions of workers, male and female, redundant. Jobs would be specialised, highly skilled and part-time. The conservative estimate of family life suggested that Daddy, for instance, would be at home most of the time; unless he was in the pub or at the football match. Possibilities not to be dismissed too lightly, reminded Mary. Mammy would have labour-saving devices which eye had not seen nor ear heard, and even the advertising wizards would have trouble enough inventing new gadgets to keep her occupied at home. Everyone would be much better educated.

However, it was Mary's description of less conservative prophecies of future family life that brought wrath on the heads of all of us. This claimed that family life would disappear, to be replaced by some version of the commune. Children would be considered too precious to be brought up, as they now were, in whatever haphazard fashion the amateurs who bred them hit upon. Those entrusted with the young would be well-trained and suited to the task, natural parents or otherwise.

This is the talk that curdles blood in a culture such as ours, which upholds the nuclear family as the most sacred of all social institutions. Nevertheless, recalled Mary, up to a hundred years ago children were reared in the extended family. In the last two generations the family had dwindled to the primary parent-children unit. Now, for the first time in history, children were growing up in the suburban environment, where the only adult they saw apart from the postman and the breadman was mother. It was the first time women had been so isolated from other adults, restricted for eight to ten hours daily to the company of little children. It was the first time that men had to travel long distances to work, to large factories and offices where they were increasingly only one cog in a multitude, at tasks where the end product was more remote and less personally meaningful than ever before.

And what was so wonderful, dared Mary Maher, about contemporary Irish society? She referred to the increase in crime, alcoholism, mental illness. If women was about anything, it was about women co to change those aspects of society that were im relevant to them, "issue by issue, with an eye towa what's going to become of their grand-daughters."

It was when Mary Maher went on television to express these views, on a "Late Late Show" one Saturday night in October 1970, that she really ignited a storm. Mary Kenny, Nell McCafferty and I were on the same show. Typical of the way the researchers set up these events, we women were brought out as wild bulls to face popular matadors with all the weight of public opinion on their side. The middle-aged Irish bachelor is a sure subject of popularity, considered a grand fellow, admired for having so far slipped the noose of marriage, with a usually inappropriate aura of being God's gift to women, a touch of "catch-me-if-you-can". And tonight, the star attraction was a decidedly non-feminist bachelor from Tipperary, John McConville, flanked by the newscaster Dermot Mullane and the ever-lovely Shirley Temple Black, she being a living example of just how far a nice woman can make it without all this silly women's lib.

One can see now that this item of the show was to be one of those circus numbers in which feminists would be deliberately baited and then bashed for answering back. At Mass the following morning, people would raise their eyes to Heaven at us outrageous, unattractive females. In Ireland, where it is considered outrageous to be sexually attractive, to be *unattractive* is among the worst sins, undermining as it does the whole quality of Irish life. The most popular TV panellist is either a virginal-looking sexpot or a sexy-looking virgin. We were bound to be discredited ...

From my later experience as a researcher, I can guess how the show would have been shaped. First of all, Ambassador Shirley Temple Black would have been "on offer". Good television for Ireland. Then someone on the team would have suggested getting some of the women's libbers to come on with her, and John McConville would have been added to the mix. Now the balance was wrong, so you'd need another man, and Dermot Mullane would be cast in the rôle. Both men were *delightfully* provocative on the subject of women, and of course Shirley Temple was *utterly* charming and reasonable. It all worked like a dream. We rose to the bait.

It was a hell of a night. Mary Maher really laid her head on the chopping-block when she suggested that the state should take an interest in the needs of motherhood and child-care. Worse, she said that every child born should be supported by the state.

The following Wednesday a thoughtful piece on the current phase of women's liberation appeared in the *Irish Times,* written by Maeve Binchy. Without ever striking any dramatic postures, Maeve has always been a quiet champion of women's rights, and both her bestselling novel, *Light A Penny Candle,* and her award-winning television play, *Deeply Regretted By* ... give a sensitive portrayal of women's lives. The TV play examined the tragedy of divorce Irish style; it was about the English family of an Irish emigrant who has a wife at home in Ireland, and dies leaving neither wife aware of the existence of the other. The situation could be treated as farce; Maeve makes it into a gentle tragedy.

Back in 1970, her article remarked how slow to be heard were the voices of women's liberation in Ireland, apart from some social clubs, associations and unions that tried pathetically to win a better deal for some women in some limited areas of their lives. Real liberation, said Maeve, meant not just bra-burning but above all answering back: "It has a lot to do with the fear of challenging what they understand and finding something new to put in its place ... Everyone will agree it is monstrous to have women architects being offered hundreds of pounds less a year than their male counterparts by the Board of Works, to have female cleaners scrubbing offices for less than male cleaners." An equally liberated sex-life for men and women was impossible in a society where more men emigrated and spinsters abounded. To catch one of the few men about, one had better play it safe, don the cash-mere sweater, the row of pearls and the demure look. Marriage, she conceded, might be a boring ship, but it was one of the few ocean-going vessels around.

Interviewing women for their reactions to last Saturday's "Late Late Show", Maeve found few that were willing to be quoted and even fewer worth quoting. They were not enthusiastic about women's lib. One woman declared that it was about as relevant as a race relations board in Kilkenny. Men fumed that it was a wonder there were not more deserted wives if we were an example of Irish womanhood. Mary Maher's remarks about every child being entitled to state support was apparently seen as strik-ing against the very roots of family life and masculine authority. It threatened not only the patriarch's power over his children, but over their mothers as well. It was easy to see that the surest way of maintaining women as dependent beings, of maintaining their oppression, would be by women themselves, just as slavery is always main-tained by those who absorb their masters' view of them, believing it right and natural that they be enslaved.

Letters to the Editor came pouring in: "Does she really want a society where promiscuous women cease taking precautions and have child after child for financial gain?" asked a lady from Tullamore, unaware perhaps that "pre-cautions" were unavailable at that time to the vast majority of Irish women who needed to take them. "Does she wish the father of too many children to desert his wife so that the state will maintain her?" Alas, many Irish fathers had already found this solution to their virility, nor was the state concerning itself with abandoned wives. She was all for women's liberation if it helped widows and the unmarried mother (who she stated was rarely a promis-cuous woman), helping her to keep her baby with state support, but these were things men wanted too, she said. Personally, my researches failed to uncover such a male. None wrote to the papers. Nor did one appear on tele-vision. However, my heart went out to this correspondent when she revealed what many older women must have felt

— still feel — which was that they were being dismissed as wasted, beyond hope, by women's liberation. "Didn't we rear you, for a start?" she demanded.

Indeed they did. I always felt a bit guilty about not inviting my own mother along to Gaj's. I used to think she might understand, had a lot to offer. But nobody invited her mother. It wasn't exactly an unspoken rule, it just didn't happen. Fear of being discovered at what one was doing, of being coaxed into compromise. Looking back, it was as impossible as asking one's mother to play blind man's buff or one of those "wicked" kissing games one played at parties when I was an adolescent.

One's mother belongs to the world one wants to change, to the self one fears becoming. And the mother's status in a man's world awakens questions. In *Of Woman Born,* Adrienne Rich writes of that complex relationship between mother and daughter: "The loss of the daughter to the mother, the mother to the daughter is the essential female tragedy ... A mother's victimization also mutilates the daughter who watches her for clues as to what it means to be a woman." Rich examines matrophobia, estrangement from the mother, and pronounces it symptomatic of the daughter's unsatisfied need of mothering. Few women growing up in a patriarchal society can feel mothered enough; the power of mothers is simply too restricted. And it is through the mother that patriarchy teaches the small female her proper expectations. "Many daughters live in rage at their mothers for having accepted, too readily and passively, whatever comes."

A man may sometimes give his daughter the ego support that he withholds from his wife, says Adrienne Rich. A male teacher can nurture a woman student while throttling his own wife and daughters. "Men have been able to give power, support, and certain forms of nurture, as individuals, when they choose; but the power is always stolen power, withheld from the mass of women in patriarchy." Favoured women — Daddy's girls — are often bewildered by the passivity and powerlessness of other women. Thus nourished by the father, they identify with male power and do not fear ending up as powerless as their mothers. Discrimination against women has not hurt them, so they do not fight against it.

My own confirmation as a woman, the woman I am and not the woman I "should be" has come from other women, especially from women in that group of the 'seventies, the Gaj's group. But whether we can pass this on to our daughters remains to be seen. Again I quote Adrienne Rich: "Until a strong line of love, confirmation, and example stretches from mother to daughter, from woman to woman across the generations, women will still be wandering in the wilderness."

And yet we talked a lot about our mothers, about their lives, their experience, their hopes for us. The rejection of mothers, I learned there, even the part rejection or imagined rejection is insurmountable. Some women spend their lives looking for the ideal mother, demanding it from husbands, lovers. Others mother everybody, marry babies only to realise (if at all) that they are hooked on giving what they have most wanted. One woman in the group turned on me angrily once: "I know I want mothering, but don't smother me. That's *your* power trip." Somebody suggested a Mother's Night, but it was dropped. Somebody said her mother wouldn't get along with anybody else's mother. So we excluded our mothers, but they were there, in all of us. If only ...

"If, don't give me ifs," someone used to say to me years ago, translating from the original Yiddish, "if Granny had balls she'd be your Grandpa." So we didn't invite our mothers to our liberation meetings, our consciousness-raising sessions, our plans to change the world.

Two Dublin social workers, Nora O'Connor and Maeve Kennedy, wrote to "Women First" in the *Irish Times* about the appalling treatment of women in Ireland: "When Ireland got her freedom in 1916, apparently they interpreted it to mean that it only referred to men. 1916 never happened for Irish women. It was only a transfer of domination from one authority to another." They set out the many glaring injustices against women which they met every day of their working lives. Some scandals, like the unfair treatment of married women under the tax code, or the miserable allowances for widows, were already notorious. But other allegations were new and fairly astonishing, such as their revelation that they frequently came across cases where a married man brought another woman in to live in the family home (which was, of course, "his" property). The two writers, naturally, demanded joint home ownership, as well as legislation compelling men to give two-thirds of their earnings to their families.

Another letter to "Women First" in the aftermath of that infamous "Late Late Show" gave hearty encouragement to the women's movement. Those men would not have said what they did if the women were black, for fear of being branded racist. What women's liberation really demanded was that women be given a fair deal, a practical choice, not just either/or: either stay single and work, or get married and stay at home. And as for methods, this correspondent asked, when looking for attention "isn't bra-burning preferable to a bomb or hi-jacking?"

The author of the letter was Phil Moore, who has since made an impressive commitment to the women's movement as chairwoman of the Women's Political Association. Over the years, the WPA has backed women candidates in Irish elections, endeavoured to educate the electorate. Taking over where the suffragettes left off, the first slogan of the Women's Political Association was "Why Not A Woman?". Later, there was no longer any need for that question, the new slogan enquired confidently: "Who's Your Woman?"

That "Women First" column contained some pretty sharp contributions. From a woman who knew her onions as well as her status sufficiently well to sign herself merely "M.O'F" came the following:

"Some say that we are already liberated in Ireland. We don't need this Women's Liberation gimmick. But to-night in each of a thousand homes a woman will sit alone, because himself is gone out for his nightly fun with the boys and there is no one else to look after the children ...

Is she liberated on Friday nights when she is offered what is probably one-third of his wages to cover all her household expenses and feed a family of eight, while the rest is securely pocketed for boozing and gambling purposes? Did they liberate her when she was a girl and the nuns taught her Latin and Domestic Science in an all-female institution ...? Was she liberated when she finally got a job and she worked as hard and as long and as conscientiously as the young fellow at the next desk or the next machine and she received 60% of his wages in return? Did they liberate her when they took her hard-earned ten bob at the door of the dance-hall week after week and in return allowed her the privilege of standing like a piece of merchandise in a gaily-coloured display, to be assessed and inspected by prospective buyers who expect an excellent return for their own ten bob investment?

"They tell her she is liberated ... she has a home and a family and her biological urges are satisfied, and after all, what more could a woman want? Perhaps they are right. Any well-behaved sow with a new litter of bonhams would agree."

That anonymous awareness, frustration, bitterness was what drove the women's movement forward in Ireland in the years that followed. Even if they never wrote a letter, women's support was felt. They stopped you in the street and said: "I couldn't speak up for women the way you do, but I'm with you and I think you are great." Once such a woman pressed a fiver into my hand in Grafton Street and sped on. I didn't know what to do with the fiver and kept it in a separate part of my hand-bag for weeks until a travelling woman who looked sick, was pregnant and had a child in her arms begged from me. I gave her the fiver, imploring her to spend even one pound on herself. She'd had her first child at sixteen and was carrying her seventeenth, six dead.

Of course there was plenty of support that was far from anonymous, but I was always deeply touched by the idea of all the nameless women recognised in Carolyn A. Krill's song, "Speak For Me Too":

I can't tell you who I am, I have no name,
Call me weak, call me tired, call me old.
I am frightened by the label;
want to speak but I'm not able.
When you speak, will you speak for me too?

There we were, a bunch of mad feminist women, describing a colour the "decent people of Ireland" claimed they could not see. We were the ones supposed to be out of step, despised, ridiculed, the butt of that awful, derisive, ever-present Irish laughter described by Shaw in *John Bull's Other Island*. How could you respond to the violence of that jeering, invalidating laughter? That's what made those other "normal" voices so sweet to the senses. They were the voices of the plain women of Ireland, the wives and mothers, the acceptable women who could not be put down as harridans or lesbians or left-overs from the marriage markets. And they were supporting us.

Those voices, in some sense, represented our mothers. The question of motherhood was never far below the surface in the founder group. Well-behaved sows we might not be, but we had had our litters. Of the women who figured prominently at the time, only two or three were single. Máire Woods had six children at the time, and later two more, "in spite," as one young woman put it, "of being a doctor and being able to do something about contraception." Máirín Johnston, Margaret Gaj, myself and Mary Maher had eleven children between us. (Not that that is any claim to fame. I was once in the company of six women with sixty-nine children between them). Still, we were mothers.

Mary Maher, who produced two baby daughters, Maeve and Nora, in the same year, was an ideal person to bring women's liberation to Irishwomen. As she talked and wrote, she struggled to hold on to her own identity, against the same odds as most Irishwomen of her time. She had the same "handicap" as anyone else: an Irish husband, Des Geraghty (to whom I apologise for calling him a handicap, trusting he knows what I mean), Irish in-laws, a traditionally Irish Catholic background in the States. It was from Mary Maher's lips that I first heard Article 41 of the Constitution of Ireland, which recognises that "by her life within the home, woman gives to the State a support without which the common good cannot be achieved. The State shall therefore endeavour to ensure that mothers shall not be obliged by economic necessity to engage in labour to the neglect of their duties in the home." (Given this commitment to the institution of marriage, I've always wondered why the state doesn't do something real and unambivalent about alcoholism, which represents a charging army against family life. That might be more useful than banning divorce in the Constitution).

Mary Maher's Irish background in Chicago was borne out by her parents' ready acceptance that she would go to live in Dublin. They were grateful for small mercies; she could have suggested worse. London, maybe. They thought that going to Dublin was safe, like going to live in a church. From the beginning, Mary found it "really more like living in a pub". She arrived in 1965, and was immediately enchanted. She was on three months' probation with the *Irish Times* at fifteen pounds a week, and went to the pub with the boys every day after work. She loved it, for although Chicago was not an emancipated place for women, it was OK to take a glass or two before going home and then maybe a movie with a pizza afterwards. Perhaps, Mary thought, the after-work drinks would lead to something else, but in Ireland they invariably led to more of the same. Irishmen then, more than now, do not go to the pictures with girls unless they are going with them seriously, "doing a line", as they say. So Mary stayed in the pub where it didn't rain.

She was often the only female in the place, whether it was the old Pearl Bar in Fleet Street or the Bailey in South Anne Street. Brendan Behan held insulting court in O'Neill's of Merrion Row, around the corner from Leinster House, where the types were political, *Gaelgeoirs* and civil servants. She was delighted at being one of the gang, felt a sense of camaraderie — which proves that she didn't know enough about the Irish way of doing things. Where were the other women? Nor did she miss the female company. Eventually, of course, wake-up time came for this sleeping beauty. It was the night the boys decided to smuggle her into a shebeen "for a bit of gas". The drill was perfect. The barman, who hated women, threw out the keys in a match-box to the pavement below. Everyone made their way up the stairs, but he spotted Mary amongst the men and whispered vehemently "No women allowed". Since he had the power not to allow any of the others either, the lads wished her a safe journey home.

Now Mary went in search of a girl-friend, or at least female company: "When the Women's Movement in Ireland complains now of women not in public life, I must stifle my memory lest I appear too ancient and irrelevant a crone; but it wasn't that long since they were entirely invisible." She found the women in tea-rooms, the sort of place where a girl could meet her friends for beans on toast for three shillings and sixpence each. The regular garb was a tweed suit worn with a black polo-necked jumper from October to March. The earnings of these nice girls kept them modest in dress as well as every other way. They indulged themselves in the pictures with a huge bag of sweets, window-shopped, and lived with their parents if they were Dubliners. Girls coming from all over the country to work in the capital lived four or five in places called flats. They were partitioned bits of fine old Dublin houses, always small and high-ceilinged. Mary found Irish girls warm and joyous friends, cynical, intelligent, "dry and philosophical about their plight and frequently able to outwit it by achieving the impossible." Now Mary saw Ireland not as the land of poets and scholars but as a dreadful country for women. There was no mention of such a hope as equality. You did what you were expected to do. You applied your education to snare a man and marry him, and since men spent most of their time at football or hurley matches or in the pub ...

She recalls the rugby hop, the Saturday night dance at the rugby club, where one went to get a fella. Three hours of cosmeticking were pre-ritual to the dance. She wrote about the agony of it all in a memorable column. The hall was full of girls, lovely, bedecked, three deep along the walls and nary a lad in sight. Then it was closing-time and the boys wafted in on a breeze of Guinness. The dance was over at midnight, so that an hour after the fellows arrived it was all over, the homegoing arrangements having been made. That was the weekly ritual of mating, like a Saturday laxative, and the amazing thing was that everyone went back for more. It was the same when my vintage of girls went to the dances, but then there was absolutely *no* other opportunity for mating attempts. Most fellows and girls met their mates in that awful way in Ireland, and still do to an extent, but I remember at eighteen being amazed that I had managed to "get" a husband outside the tyranny of the Saturday night ritual in the rugby club.

The cattle mart of the dance hall was nature's triumph over all, because it got the sexes together, but with what a clash and at what a price. The women were resentful of having to work so hard to be noticed, the men were terrified of women, preferring the pub. Both were chaste and chased in this convoluted way until they trapped each other. "It was a social system which virtually ensured the enduring enmity of the sexes and guaranteed that friendships on an equal basis, let alone liaisons of a meaningful nature, were unachievable. And since that kind of equality is the kind that means most to most women for most of their lives, the system set discrimination in concrete moulds," said Mary.

But then along came the lounge bars, and the girls abandoned their tea rooms. Here you could stalk the prize on its own territory. The lounge was like a river full of trout, lively and shimmery and apparently oblivious to the threat of the hook, but nonetheless slippery for all that. Many's the woman who found a mate in a lounge bar more easily lost than the thirst she developed en route. But that, says Mary, was the beginning of the social emancipation of Irishwomen, a beginning of the end of Irishmen, single or married, having pubs to themselves, hide-aways, homes from homes where being sociable meant being with the boys. She emphasises that the entry of Irishwomen to pubs must not be overlooked as we remember equal pay, law reform, Family Planning Centres and Well Woman Clinics.

The amazing advance, says Mary, is that nowadays Irishwomen often prefer their own company to that of men. And yet, it wasn't through meeting other women that she was to discover her feminine self, but through giving birth to two daughters. The fact that her involvement with the women's movement coincided with the birth of her two daughters had an amazing impact on her, took her years to figure out. The truth was that she had never anticipated them — had assumed, although hardly consciously, that she would have boys: robust, aggressive sons. She had three older brothers, her husband was one of a family of five boys, and she was, she says, scared to death of bringing up girls. She put the thought straight out of her mind throughout the first pregnancy. How many women are scared of their own femininity. In 1969, Mary Maher identified with the masculine world of power and achievement.

Now, she thinks that shows how screwed up she was about the feminine-masculine identity thing, and how ambivalent she was about her relationship with her mother. It wasn't just that girls had a much harder time in the world, it was that she felt frightened of what kind of a mother she would be to a girl. She had negative feelings about being female herself, being like her mother, and was afraid to confront them.

There is that bind again: to be like the mother and fail, or reject one's mother in oneself and feel the awful sense of betrayal. "I promised myself I'd be different when I had a daughter of my own." With Mary, as with lots of other women, the very thought of reversing rôles, being the mother of a daughter, was not allowed to surface. She was at that point from which so many women never move in relation to her mother, the point at which it is impossible to see that Woman in our lives as she was before she became Mother, as she is apart and in spite of being Mother. Instead of searching that out, we accept the blurb,

262

the Mother's Day mush, the cosy, unthreatening part of what they are for us.

"I often felt I probably would not have become pregnant promptly again had the first one been a boy. Not on a conscious level, but ingrained, was the conviction, the old cliché, that families should start with boys, that sons were more important," says Mary, and I remember that when my Adam was born, apart from thinking I had done something great, I had the awareness that I had done something exactly right. First born, a son. Not that I'd have sent a girl back, as they say, or even been aware that I could have gone one better, but that feeling was there.

Fortunately Mary never had a negative response to either baby once born; the old bonding was a pretty powerful experience. "Anyway," she says, "having the two small emphatically female babies made me confront a lot of what was in myself and forced me to work things out, sometimes on the hop. I had to look at how much in my own background had reinforced the conviction that females were inferior, and I had to work out the balance between the two worlds I had grown up with, wanting both: the 'feminine' world — I wanted to have children, wanted that nurturing rôle, the reward — and the 'masculine' world, being taken as a serious person, having personal work to do and goals to achieve quite apart from children or family. I often used to half-laugh, half-cry at the contradictions in myself. I would dress the two of them up in the absolute pinkest lace I could find and then militantly ensure that they had non-sexist toys to play with. I wanted both for them as for myself. It took me a while to say right, that's what they are entitled to.

"I have found it fascinating and rewarding to talk to my daughters about feminism as they grow up and while I'm sure I've made mistakes I feel a real surge of joy sometimes when I think they will *never* [her emphasis on *never* is total, joyous] face the same conflicts as my generation did, that they assume equality and have a natural confidence in it when so many women had to battle their way there, before."

Mary sees the Women's Movement as having been invaluable to her in this personal way. Had she been the mother of two girls twenty years ago, being the way she was, with all the same influences at work on her life, she knows she would have made a much worse job of it. Would never have begun to resolve the difficulties. Would not have even known how to name them.

Mary Maher is now "Mother" of the *Irish Times* chapel of the National Union of Journalists, a position hitherto known as "Father". When she asked a colleague if she should insist on being called Mother rather than the established Father, it was decided that she would address any man as "Sister" who called her by the old title. Mary now sees the way ahead as through an equality movement rather than a women's movement.

14
THE LAST DECADE

The public resignations and the quieter departures of other members of the Founder Group did not upset the rest of us as much as might have been supposed. For one thing, we were unaware of what was happening — the beginning of the end of us as a group — or the reasons. We had our problems and they seemed more real than the petty accusations, the childish insistence that everything could be sorted out to please everybody.

After the Mansion House everything had happened so fast that we were, literally, lost in confusion. The anticipation had been better than the realisation. Gone was the headiness and now there was frustration and dissatisfaction, bringing a sliding sense of anti-climax, even failure. Above all, collectively and individually, we were exhausted. And, I believe we were too ignorant of the workings of group energy to understand that things were working out predictably.

We had done what came naturally to a radical group so full of media people. We'd broken the news. We'd told Ireland about the women's movement. We'd turned women on. We'd revealed the underground anger in women's lives, we'd blown the cover. We'd been like the four-and-twenty blackbirds baked in the pie and when the pie was opened the birds began to sing and wasn't that a dainty dish to set before patriarchy? Think of all the singing at various pitches, in orchestral chorus now and imagine how it was, inside that pie, before we broke that crust of silence with our shrillness.

A garda whom I met in the Wicklow hills recently, said: "I thought ye lot were going to blow it at one stage. Starting the women's movement was important but it looked, for a while, that you were going to put off the very people you needed. Women have come a long way since then. What happened to the original group? Why did you break up?"

We "broke up" because a mass movement could not have been built into an autocratic organisation, a national women's club, without fatally diluting the blood of that movement. The basic difference between a movement and an organisation still isn't realised by so many women unconsciously trying to replace one authoritarian system with another. An organisation is task-orientated, a movement is person-orientated. Organisations can and do thrive within the women's movement, but the movement itself cannot be structured within an organisation.

In her brilliant pamphlet, *The Tyranny of Structurelessness,* Jo Freeman pinpoints the limitations of "leaderless" groups. Contrary to what we would like to believe, she pointed out, there is no such thing as a structureless group, because the idea of structurelessness only prevents the formation of formal structures, not informal ones. Unstructured groups may be very effective in getting women to start talking about their lives, said Freeman, but they weren't very good for getting things done. Certainly, what happened in the Gaj's group when we wanted to organise an activity was exactly as Freeman described: friendship groups became the main means of organisational activity. So you got élitism. Structurelessness also spawned the star system. The public is conditioned to look for spokespeople, while the movement itself has not worked out how to express its views. And so stars are created, rather than elected, out of the structureless group. Women known to the public, or who spoke up when pressed, were labelled "stars" of the movement. Most undemocratic. But by purging a sister who had exhibited stardom, the movement lost whatever control it might have had over her; she then became free to commit all the individualistic sins of which she had been accused. So, in a manner of speaking, the founder group was unconsciously pushed out by the other groups, now the mass of the movement, as a bunch of "stars".

Our attempt to structure our group came too late. Besides our main task was done. The movement continued, and in our different ways we were all part of it, especially on an individual basis of personal development. For instance, when Nuala Fennell said she left Women's Lib and started all over again, she didn't. With her followers she carved out a task that needed doing, and in doing it formed an organisation, AIM, which immediately became a definable part of the movement. In the same way, any woman who says "I'm not a woman's libber, but I believe in women's rights" is a sister of the movement. Her life will be affected by changing attitudes and legislation changing her own status and attitudes. Increasingly, women are making personal connective changes in their own lives, contributing to further possibilities of change. The women in the world who have not yet awakened to their right to make choices about their own lives are like sleeping beauties whose time may or may not come. Others swallow some package of women's liberation hook, line and sinker, and suffer a chronic pain in the throat. Only swallow what you can digest!

Meanwhile, the Founder Group was disintegrating. Consciousness-raising had brought individual awareness to the surface. Most of us were now faced with personal, inescapable looking-glasses. This could no longer be externalised. The cud must be chewed, no matter how the socialists decried such personal indulgence. People who change things are inevitably changed by their own thoughts and actions. It was time to deal with some changes in ourselves. We could no longer avoid looking at our personal states, sorting out our personal liberation.

As things were, a tyrannical superego, born of the movement, had begun to sound like parental nagging in many ears. We had a new boss. The silent Voice of the women's movement was capable of creating a claustrophobia as dense as we'd ever experienced before. There was the unspoken fear of not being worthy of the sisterhood. Who was being regressive or disloyal to the cause? Was I always going to dress like a Barbie Doll and make up to men? I remember telling the man in my life who had dropped me off at Gaj's, to park around the corner and I'd walk. He chuckled knowingly. It went without saying that getting there under one's own steam, preferably on the bus was in the proper spirit of things.

Much as I liked the "game", I felt uncomfortable about some of the unspoken "rules". It was made worse by the fact that one was treated as a guru by so many women outside the group, with the uncomfortable inference that one was actually liberated. Like hell I was! I'm still only pointed in the right direction.

Personally, I couldn't have borne it if I'd known the group was falling apart forever. But it happened gently. Máirín de Burca had increased responsibilities in Sinn Féin and had to drop out. Máirín Johnston, who was rumoured to have got pregnant the night of the Contraceptive Train (any woman who produced a baby within two years after the train was said to have got pregnant that night) was too content to battle for the time being. Máire Woods' husband died after a long illness. Robert Woods, the surgeon, had had terminal cancer, and Máire's courage during that time held many in awe of her. I dissolved into a state of exhaustion. I used to do that periodically until my friend Marie Berber stood over my bed one day saying: "For such an intelligent woman you can be quite dumb, can't you? D'you not *feel* yourself getting tired? Why wait until you've run yourself into the ground ...?"

And then Mary Kenny got the job in the *Evening Standard* and was off to London. That was hard to take. No matter what anyone said, no matter what her weaknesses or strengths, Mary *was* a leader. The covert structure of our structureless group had projected her in a way that would have been pretty difficult to decline even had she wished. We felt abandoned. Nell McCafferty went off to

France, but came back and joined the Fownes Street group, which dropped the word "Irish", saying it was "élitist", and modestly called itself The Women's Liberation Movement. Mary Maher was bogged down with two youngsters and determined to keep her job. Margaret Gaj's husband was sick.

There was never a last meeting in Gaj's. It was like a flower whose petals fell away, naturally, slowly, leaving the plant behind, its seed to scatter on the winds.

When it began, most of us were like Rachel in Virginia Woolf's *The Voyage Out*, awakening, forced out from the purdah of fantasy woven by society. Rachel comes to her first awareness of being a woman in a man's world.

> "So that's why I can't walk alone!"
> By this new light she saw her life for the first time a creeping hedged-in thing, driven cautiously between high walls, here turned aside, there plunged in darkness, made dull and crippled forever — her life that was the only one she had — a thousand words and actions became plain to her.
> "Because men are brutes! I hate men!" she exclaimed.
> "I thought you said you like him?" said Helen.
> "I liked him and I liked being kissed," she answered, as if that only added more difficulties to her problem.

But it is through this experience that she learns that she can be herself, be a person on her account, in spite of everything and everybody.

* * *

I was working as a free-lance journalist in 1974, mainly with the *Sunday Independent* when a vacancy occurred on the research team of the "Late Late Show". I'd often appeared on the show as a panellist and I liked Gay Byrne. I wanted the job for two reasons. First, I was going through one of those "feeling insecure" phases suffered by most free-lance writers. Not being entitled as a free-lance to sickness or holiday pay, much less a chance to doss around, can sometimes have a tendency to bring on maladies and exhaustion. The second reason was my dream of a mass outlet for my feminist missionary zeal.

Of course everyone working on the show was prepared for this zeal, especially Gay. He was, in a manner of speaking, armed to the teeth, taking me on because of my journalistic experience and "quirky way of thinking", but wary of my enthusiasm in relation to women's issues. I found Gay to be a male chauvinist, but hardly a pig. I didn't think he took myself or Pan seriously enough then, because we were women, but "pig" was far too harsh a description for a man who is decent, professional and usually good-humoured. He was often impatient with my suggestions for women's programmes, but then so were most of the team.

At that stage, not many people in RTE realised that women were here to stay. The women's movement, like any other mystifying female madness, would pass. I had to work harder to "sell" Gay a women's issue or a woman panellist (unless she was glamorous as well as a brilliant talker) than any hare-brained show-biz bit of nonsense I might dream up. Mind you, I had no difficulty getting him to present the annual Ballybunion Bachelors' Competition as a male beauty show.

The boys had to parade twice, once in their bathing trunks and then in suits. Grace O'Shaughnessy, the famous model did the commentary, giving each man's vital statistics. I added one unnamed statistic to each set of measurements. It referred to the biceps. People in the studio squirmed at their own guesswork. TV viewers meeting me during the following couple of weeks kept saying things like: "I couldn't believe you'd measured *that,* but I couldn't think what else it could be. But you wouldn't *dare.*"

But they measure breasts, don't they?

As for asking the contestants silly questions and getting predictably silly answers, I don't think many people got the point. For instance: "Will you give up working when you get married?" was too much before its time in Ireland to even raise a laugh.

And so it went on. I battled consistently at trying to get women's issues on TV, sometimes feeling quite punch-drunk, but bouncing back off the ropes to fight another round. When I feared the straight approach would fail, I tried to get around Gay — in ways too despicable to mention — but he could feel me coming with a women's lib item a mile off. He'd sigh deeply, making it clear that he was resigning himself to hearing me out, look relieved if someone else opposed the idea before he'd given his verdict. I'd be furious. This was like a boys' club, I'd rave, women had a right to be represented on the "Late Late". Besides, weren't they more than half the viewing population? "How come they don't want to know, Junie?" he'd ask, sure of his thrust, "how come they switch off?" Sometimes, he'd make an act of being about to do me a big favour, because he was sorry for me: "OK, find me a woman for this item." I'd try, but often there simply was not a woman around who was expert and articulate enough on the particular subject. When I'd find a woman, half joking, wholly in earnest he'd ask: "What does she look like?" Periodically, he'd throw out an order to the team to get some glamour. "We need a gorgeous woman. Come on gang, there must be some talent out there ..." I'd fume.

"Find me someone like Arianna Stassinopoulos, June," he said once and my head jerked up in time to catch him straightening his grin. When I had appeared on the same show with Arianna Stassinopoulos, author of *The Female Woman*, I'd had to work so hard at controlling my rage, frustration and impotence that traces of it stayed with me like a hypnotic suggestion. My frustration was with the beautiful Greek's perfect impersonation of the female woman, a carefully co-ordinated drag act which left Máirín Johnston and myself as the ugly sisters. In having the education to write a real live scholarly book — I had to keep looking up words and references — I knew that she had enjoyed male advantages, that she was utterly atypical of her countrywomen. A graduate of Cambridge, she was now doing postgraduate work and had completely distanced herself from the life context of the vast majority of "female women", whose natural happiness was being threatened, she claimed, by the women's movement. My impotence was caused by the fact that I did not have the educational information to counterattack. Hers was a male chauvinist trip, a projection of the ultimate double standard: this is the way *you* should live, but it's not good enough for me.

Viewers who hadn't read the book, naturally were delighted with her feminine ways. She said all the things they wanted to hear, looked the way a woman *should* look, and created a "beautiful victim" aura with a wave of her slender, much-tended hand, a glance of deliberately ill-suppressed distaste at irrelevancies when she was reminded of the facts of women's lives. Watching, Nuala Fennell told me later that my face was a study in conflicting emotions. I was angry, but determined to recognise her in sisterhood. It wasn't going to be easy. She castigated women's libbers as man-haters, woman-haters, child-haters. She claimed that radical change was being forced on women who were perfectly happy as they were, which drew an angry growl from Mairin: "You have the arrogance of your class!" Miss Stassinopoulos went on to accuse the women's movement of visiting our thwarted hangups on "normal" women. Some of us, she delicately suggested, were lesbian. Could I possibly be forgiven for disgracing myself then, right at the end of the programme, with no chance to recant, by lazily remarking something along the lines that homosexuality was hardly a new idea for Greeks? No, whatever the remark, whatever its context and provocation, it was racist, prejudiced and sexist. Only one viewer wrote in to complain.

During International Women's Year, 1975, I "found" Gay the columnist and TV personality Anna Raeburn. "Well done, Junie," he said of this brilliant, sensitive woman, "I wonder does she fancy me?" He found Lady Miranda Iveagh irresistible because "she's so beautiful and nice and soft and approachable ..." Studying his tastes would give a researcher an excellent idea of the type of woman sure of a chance on the "Late Late Show". I was always on the look-out for women who reminded me of the women he liked, such as Eimer Philbin Bowman (a friend of the Byrne family and one of the Gaj's group), his beautiful and perfect secretary Maura Connolly, and his wife, the red-haired Kathleen Watkins, multi-talented and maternal. The women he liked were by no means all confined to the ladylike stereotype moulded through generations of Irish convents. However, the dropped eyelash, the virginal giggle, the faint flush of pink to the cheek were never lost on Gay. Like any Irishman, docility came high on his list of womanly qualities, but he also responded favourably to vaguely covert high-spiritedness. And of course, talent.

"There is nothing so disillusioning as to be talking to a beautiful woman and have her, in the course of conversation, deliver herself of an appalling crudity," he once told me. He hated being reminded that a woman had bodily functions. Once I said: "Look, I'll settle down to this discussion after I've nipped out to the lavatory ..." He flinched and said "Charming!" It's only worth mentioning because that's the way celibate religious teachers educated Irish fellows to think about women, as a different species, "dangerous cattle" to be avoided if possible, the company of whom led one into terrible moral danger. Eventually, one would marry, perhaps, but naturally to a girl who didn't mention lavatories.

The most professional person I ever met in my life, Gay was unstinting in his appreciation of achievers in any area, of either sex. As a boss, he was ruthless. I learned soon that I was mere fodder for the show. I often felt cannibalised. Every scrap of oneself was expected to go into his show. "It's only an old television programme," I'd tease him. He never thought for a moment that I could be serious.

Often there would be no pleasing him. He'd pick on

everyone in turn, have us picking on each other. I'd gradually learned a bit, through reading and watching, about what happens to people in groups. But Gay appeared to be totally unconscious of the undercurrents, the group energy. He wouldn't admit that a team member had been cast as scapegoat or favourite. He'd set us against each other sometimes, and leave us to fight it out between us, as if he knew somewhere in a remote corner of his brain that the frustrated energy would somehow be driven into the show.

Often, he was like a Christian Brother of the nasty type Irishmen have described to me, merciless, unreasonable, relentless in his attack on anyone who fell short. The group structure was simple and rigid: "I'm the boss, always right. *You* deliver." A researcher could have spent a whole week on an item and made complicated arrangements, but if Gay got a hunch or something better, he'd cancel the whole thing.

As a friend, he was as gentle as he could be tough, as understanding as he could be unreasonable, accepting, affectionate and loyal, the sort who'd do you a favour behind your back. When I'd made some sort of cock-up in my personal life of the kind for which I have an unswerving talent, he'd say, loud and fond: "I told you, didn't I warn you! What are you, Junie?" "A fool," I'd have to answer, because he'd keep asking until I did.

As time went by, I could see the attitude of Ireland's number 1 media man change towards women. The letters and calls to his daily radio show, he told me in an interview for *IT* magazine, had brought it home to him that there were an awful lot of extremely bright, alert, intelligent, sound women in the country who in terms of sensitivity and "moxy" were far in advance, generally, of men. He realised that so many of these women must be married to "utter dolts, who are rude, ill-mannered, brutish". He shivered at the thought that had he been a woman he might be waking up to the awful truth that "lying beside me is this brutish dolt that really I am so far ahead of ..." Gay was never so much anti-women's movement as "anti-switch-off". But he told me: "you felt so keenly about these things that I felt nothing would satisfy you, but that we do two hours on women's affairs every Saturday night."

One Tuesday morning we were having our weekly planning meeting. The mood of these meetings depended entirely on how the show had gone on the previous Saturday night. If things had gone well, then the team would confidently offer ideas for items or personalities. After a disappointing show, we knew what to expect. Such anticipation brought out the worst according to one's personality; each team member would become cuter, slyer, more defensive, explosive, or talkative. Some dirty linen had been washed in conference, knuckles rapped, and I was sounding off about women again when Tony Boland, casting director of the Department of Light Entertainment, who supplied musical items to the show, interrupted furiously: "I'm fed up feeling guilty for having a mickey!" Gay studied the papers in front of him. Another man murmured: "So am I." Pan Collins looked from Tony to me and back again, sympathetic to both of us. Dammit, how did he think I felt about being a woman in this boys' club? But the remark, from such an unexpected source as Tony, stung. Was that all I was accomplishing, forcing someone into an uncontrolled display of vulnerability?

I was a crank among cranks in RTE. It's extraordinary how many different kinds of cranks there were in RTE, all tolerated, but they were either men, or women embracing male philosophies. A feminist, in my day there, wasn't just a crank, she was a menace, a screamer, too obviously a wall-banger to listen to. RTE always calls to mind an experience I had on an Indian railway station. There was no sign of the train and I'd drunk three or four hot cups of tea to keep out the chill, surprising after a hot day. I had to find a women's room. I searched the platform, asked a couple of Indian women feeding their children, but they knew no English. I crossed the railway bridge, up steep iron steps, still not finding a place for women, and came back to my own side of the station again. I asked a man of about thirty years: "Where is the bathroom for ladies?" knowing that was how an Indian woman would phrase the request. He pondered and then said, "Follow me, it will be fine."

He led me to a place marked in Hindi: "Men's Rest Room". Desperate as I was, I drew back, but the Indian encouraged me, a practical, kindly air about him. I followed him into a large room in which men lay about on couches, sat cross-legged on the floor and looked up from their dozing or reading and withdrew their gazes again, disinterested. The air had a sharp, yet not unfamiliar smell reminding me of the steam coming from under the bread-man's horse, long ago in Dublin. The air sharpened and cut at the back of my tongue but I went on, following my Indian escort, trusting but nervous.

We entered the other end of the room where there were cubicles on either side, men standing towards the walls in between cubicles, their backs to us and my guide opened a half-door. Relievedly, behind the bolted boards, I squatted over the latrine and glancing up saw a dark head over the wall beside me, staring straight ahead. He departed before me. I left the closet and found my escort waiting nearby. With an almost imperceptible nod of his head, he invited me to follow him. Soon, through the heavy air, we came out on the station again: "Thank you very much," I said, "it was kind of you to take the trouble."

He bowed: "No problem," and smiled.

Encouraged, I asked: "Why is there no room for women?" *Now* there was a problem. He could not understand my question, looked vaguely uneasy, backed away, his hands joined together in courteous salutation.

RTE had a "Ladies", but not much space for women. I visualise our national TV station as an enormous men's room, into which a few women have sneaked out of dire necessity. But a question like mine to the Indian elicits an uneasy shrug. Things have improved since, but I recall, in 1975, finding myself sitting in the canteen with some big shot from the accounts department and having him explain to me, without the subject having been broached by anyone, why equal pay for women was a crazy idea. No country could afford it. Besides, how could wives look up to husbands if they knew women could earn as much as them?

It was about that time I wrote a four-part script on women and the women's movement for the late Jack White, then Controller of Programmes. It was a profile of Irishwomen's lives, and the beginnings of change, strung through with song, poetry, discussion. There was a head-scarfed elderly woman on top of a bus, a little girl pushing a pram, a working wife. Jack, Lord rest him, held the scripts — named "As Time Goes By" after my favourite song — in his hand and said: "Well done. Excellent really, but a bit science fiction?" I was paid for them, but they were never used.

One script was about women as portrayed through advertising. RTE's code of advertising practice still offers no protection against sexist insults. Nor does the Advertising Standards code. Women are open season in the world of Irish advertising. Says an executive of a major advertising company: "They don't even realise they are being insulted. The most insulting ads still sell the most products, whether women like you buy them or not." His own children are watching TV now, and he's begun to listen more interestedly to my views on the subject. "We shouldn't let them watch so much TV", he said one day.

He's aware that the innocence of childhood is under threat. Meanwhile, he's got stuff to sell. Some of the ads put across by his company are sinister in their portrayal of sexual rôles, irresponsibly conditioning children for the benefit of trade. You can actually write ads that don't drag anybody down, but who cares enough to bother?

Advertising copywriters script away the wonder and openness of childhood, tying its perceptions up in knots. It's hard to forgive. They know what they are doing. Through these cynical TV images, children learn false distinctions between girl and boy, man and woman. Their natural growth towards personhood is stunted by brain-washing. Clearly, the ads show, the best is to be a man because then one calls the shots, belongs to the right caste. It's good being a "lady" too, because *we* know how to please — which is just as well because if you happen to be a girl you realise soon enough that there is an awful lot of pleasing to be done, of one kind or another. Television insists that mothers exist for the sole purpose of giving pleasure. Mother does not exist in her own right. Pleasure exists through Mother. Mother *is* Pleasure. Later, the growing boy will meet lesser Pleasures who dispense Fun. The sources of Fun are beautiful young women who appreciate a fellow's perfect choice of chocolate biscuit, beer or car. Naturally, these young women are of a different type to the real Pleasure. For a start, they don't have voices as sustaining and comforting as warm breast milk. But they will learn.

The boy learns that he is in the direct line of pleasure. There's a world of it out there, promised by females of all ages, dying (literally) to please him. The girl identifies with a "natural" ability to please, the boy with the "natural" expectation of being pleased — providing, of course, that his purchasing decisions prove his worth. The girl embraces the possibility of becoming hugely excited about white clothes for all the family, the crisis of stains on sports shorts, of less than gleaming floors. She knows, without being told, who cleans the lavatory. The sudsy conversation seeps into the recesses of her brain so that she accepts that she'll cope with all that for the rest of her life, but only, mind, if she is first successful at sorting out under-arm sniffiness and putting bounce into floppy hair.

Once, a slightly retarded twenty-year-old who helps her mother around the house, confided in me that she was inclined to worry about things. Worrying things went around and around in her head, she said.

"What sort of things?" I asked.

"Problems, you know?"

"Well, tell me one worry."

"Stains that won't come out and whites that are grey ..." she said vehemently. Her eyes widened with the drama and intensity of a TV soap commercial. She brought me to the kitchen to show me the offensive objects soaking in a basin. They looked to me like a basin of white clothes in clean water. She could not come for a walk with me. What would be the use? The worry of the clothes would be in her head. We hung them out on the line together, and I assured her they were quite perfect, but as we went indoors again, she sighed heavily: "Maybe the sun will bleach them. What soap powder do you use?"

Her brother had gone off, carefree. I don't believe the difference between their intelligence was all that relevant. Had *he* been short of the full shilling, as we say in Ireland, his anxiety would not have been rooted in the state of other people's laundry. The boy watching TV sees men go fishing, eat Yorkie bars while driving great trucks. His only concern with dirty underwear is to drop it down among the women — the floor is the handiest place — from whence it will reappear, spotless in his drawer, a triumph over "Brand X".

I'm not telling women they shouldn't wash clothes. One bit of work is as valid as another. But that type of advertising poisons. It is pornography, if your definition of porn is like mine, i.e. that there is always a victim, even albeit willing, a lesser being to be used as a beast of burden. In Ireland, few schools supply a positive programme of sex education. But every child with a TV or radio in the home gets negative sex education, of the poisoning, deadening kind that has to do with superficial things and rôle playing. It's a statement about sexuality which presents the female as an object which cleans up, cheers up and puts up.

The subtle ways by which men and women are brought to think of each other as separate species was brought home to me one morning in the "Late Late" office when a few people were discussing a film of the night before. It had been a movie about a prison, in which a man was gang-raped. The scene was terrifying, but not nearly as explicit as it might have been had the victim been a woman. Watching the film, I glanced around my living-room to find that the young men there were not merely uncomfortable, but were identifying with the raped man. Visibly shocked. The following morning, discussing the film in the office, I said: "At least that kind of scene will help men identify with the horror of being raped ..." Someone interrupted: "Ah, come off it, June, not that hobby horse ..." But John Caden, co-researcher and now a radio producer, cut in: "She's right, you know!"

I believe that television advertising, like most of the ways through which women are portrayed on that media, is a contributory factor in the ever increasing incidence of rape in Western society. It has brought to the surface a rapacious undercurrent against women, encouraging men to think of women as objects which can be "taken" in the same spirit as robbing an orchard, but with more violence because the attacker sees the victim as inferior, despicable and yet having an innate and threatening human power. In every country, social attitudes are linked to the incidence of rape. In California, London, Delhi, or Dublin, rape expresses society's regard for the female sex. Women have taken to the streets in cities all over the world to protest against violence to women. In 1978, when a massive procession of women went through the streets of Dublin in protest against rape, the organising committee, "Women Against Violence Against Women", said that they wanted it to be a women's march only. I acted as a steward on that march, and moving back and forth among the lines I came across a few men. One man in the ranks, middle-aged, the father of daughters said: "There's a lot of things I'll do if I'm told, but staying away from a march like this isn't one of them. That poor girl in Sean McDermott Street is a human being!"

"That poor girl" was aged sixteen, gang-raped by eight youths, abandoned and found by the Gardaí. She was taken to Jervis Street hospital, where it was necessary to remove one of her breasts and take out her womb. Thus salvaged, she was placed in a Dublin mental hospital.

Thousands of women marched that day, reflecting their awareness of rape as the hidden fear in their lives. A man pushing children in a wide wheeler, said to his wife alongside him, "nobody's branding me as a rapist!" I can forgive men most things, because I don't believe they realise how they oppress women. However, one thing puzzles me beyond all else. Men have fought wars for every cause under the sun and no cause at all. They have travelled to the other side of the world, uninvited, to take up arms against their brothers' oppressors. What about their sisters?

In spite of the media portrayal of women as the slave class, which doesn't appear to have changed much since I left RTE in 1978, I must admit that I enjoyed my years there, being cocooned, to a large extent, among friends in the "Late Late" office who put up with my obsessions. The best of the shows I researched there were not on women's issues, I think, because these were always fraught with such subjective tension. Nor was I the only one to handle women's issues.

Sex was another subject difficult to uncover. I did a whole two hours on sexuality once which had so little sex in it that a few years later Gay Byrne couldn't even remember we had attempted a programme on the subject. I had wrangles over bringing Joyce's Molly Bloom into an appropriate part of the show — the bit about the sexual drive in creativity — but it was considered unfit for family viewing at 10 p.m. (It must have been all those urgent ecstatic Yes's of Molly's. If one says yes to sex in Ireland, it's considered a bit much to be ecstatic). Nor was an extract from the ribald *The Midnight Court* permitted. I'd thought the bit where frustrated women put the men of Ireland on trial might contribute a bit of energy, but no. So we had a vague, obscure happening with informed, sophisticated people talking about many aspects of sexuality, even historical, and somehow sex never came into it.

I tried to get a TV show for women, writing two scripts with lists of participants, something like radio's "Women Today" with a bit of fun thrown in, but was told by one boss that I didn't realise the bother there'd be trying to get enough attractive women for a weekly women's show about various topics. After all, he reminded me, television was visual.

Nuala O'Faolain, one of RTE's few women producers,

did not get much more encouragement than that in 1982 when she made her six-part "Women Talking", presented by Doireann Ní Bhriain. It was a programme made with left-overs; left-over time from making other programmes with the outside broadcasting unit, left-over labour when the day's business was done. Location was wherever the unit happened to be. If the format was necessarily simple, it worked brilliantly. The communication between the women in these groups who gathered together by impersonal invitation in local halls was a delight. It was also probably the finest bit of consciousness-raising ever presented through the media, with *women* seemingly oblivious of the boundaries which separate them in their lives — age, marital status, class, education, urban or rural background.

"Women Talking" was given a peak-time slot. Produced by women and featuring women, it fascinated many a man who watched by default. "They talk so personally," one man in his mid-thirties told me. "Women are amazing. A group of men would never expose themselves like that." Then upon reflection he offered: "Perhaps it's because women have nothing to lose?"

In 1975, International Women's Year, the theme of which was equality, development and peace, we had quite a "jamboree", as Mary Maher put it, though not much to show at the end of it all. We reached a peak of exposure through the media. And then in 1976 one saw tears coming into people's eyes in an effort not to yawn over yet another women's issue.

1975 had produced a wonderful emergence of feminist faces, hitherto not seen or heard by the women of Ireland. They were young, brilliant, bursting with energy and commitment, and they brought home to me that the women's movement here had reached a stage where change was inevitable. There was no road back, unless as a personal choice.

Almost a caricature of the "new woman" was Anne Speed of the newly-founded Irish Women United, which contained women from several left-wing radical groups.

IWU grew out of the Fownes Street group. Anne came onto the "Late Late" via trade unionist John Caden. An active trade unionist herself, and a member of People's Democracy, Anne was involved in the women's movement since the early 'seventies. She was strongly committed to free, legal and safe contraception as a basic right for women, and is currently a member of the Women's Right to Choose Group. The slightest cue and Anne could talk and talk, rivetingly, and never repeat herself, in an unaffected Dublin accent. So many people who desire to be heard in this long-colonised land assume ruling-class English or mid-Atlantic accents. Anne was involved in the ad-hoc women's group of the Irish Transport and General Workers' Union, which adopted a "Working Women's Charter" at the 1975 annual conference. A similar charter formed the policy of Irish Women United, focussing on the rights of women workers, which included state-funded women's centres, the right to self-defined sexuality and free legal contraception. The sexual demands were thought to be brave at the time, but just as radical in Irish society was the demand for recognition of motherhood and parenthood as a social function, with state support for the socialisation of housework. The new demands of the movement in Ireland were concerned equally with women's centres, community laundries, kitchens, eating places, and self-defined sexuality. Back in 1970, not even the lesbians among us had proclaimed a woman's right to be homosexual, heterosexual, either or both.

Irish Women United contained more experienced political activists than any women's group until now, drawn from the Communist Party of Ireland, The Socialist Workers' Movement and the Movement for a Socialist Republic. They launched a contraceptive campaign, and in 1976 founded CAP, the Contraceptive Action Programme, which attempted to shake this question out of its hypocritical cloud of politicians' compromises, whereby Family Planning Clinics were allowed to "give away" free contraceptives in return for "donations", although actually "selling" the things was illegal. Scorning such deception,

CAP opened a contraceptive shop in Harcourt Street, later moving to the Dandelion Market at St. Stephen's Green, plonk in the centre of Dublin.

In the "Save the Equal Pay" Campaign in 1975, when Michael O'Leary, Labour Minister in the Coalition government, was trying to delay the new EEC legislation, the IWU brought pressure on employers rather than government, occupying the offices of the Federated Union of Employers in Fitzwilliam Place. More conventional groups bombarded the government with petitions. Thousands of us also sent letters and telegrams to Brussels to complain. The EEC saved the day; the government abolished the marriage bar, and introduced maternity leave and equal unemployment assistance. Equal pay itself does not affect the vast majority of women, who work in the lowest employment market where there is no comparison of equality to be made with men.

A year later, the IWU occupied the Forty-Foot swimming place at Sandycove Tower. I recall Nuala Fennell, who wouldn't have shared the views or tactics of that group, saying: "It's not going too far. Why should men keep the best swimming place for themselves? I remember living near the Forty-Foot and my father would take my brother to swim there and I wasn't let go." IWU also invaded the Fitzwilliam Tennis Club, closed to women. But once again, splits in ideology started to crack the movement. *Banshee,* the journal of the IWU, tried to save the life of the group, to seal the cracks between radical lesbians, left-wing socialists and mainstream feminists. Nell McCafferty, Marie McMahon and Anne Speed got out the first issues, and after that it was done by an editorial committee on a rotating basis. But the group lost the struggle with the same old bugbear, structurelessness. The dreaded word "élitist" was thrown about yet again, and IWU, which had great woman-power and talent, fell apart in 1977. Its members continue as activists in many women's groups.

By the time I went back to the "Late Late" after the summer recess of 1977, my personal life was changing so much that it seemed to be slipping beyond my grasp, or rather, racing ahead of me. It felt as if I had been moving about on a platform waiting for a train which I was not expecting for ages, when suddenly it arrived and I had to scramble myself together and board while it made threatening noises of departure.

For a start, at the end of 1976, when sounding off on a platform about my favourite topic of feminism, women and medicine, I had met a man — yes, another doctor: nothing wrong with repeating history in small details — "the rocks in whose head fitted the holes in hers," as Gore Vidal puts it. That had not quite ever happened to me before. I had been fascinated, on and off for years, by what seemed to go on in that man's head, but had not met him socially. Now, having verbally torn him to shreds in public, he offered me a lift home from the meeting. We had a drink in a pub on the way. At least he drank, I mopped the smoke out of my eyes. He talked of his own perception of the world, the need for human liberation. People walked around half-dead, he said, especially men. We were all caught up in doing, unconscious of the wonder of being. He had the contemplative's awareness of the positive activity of being, the creativity born of inner stillness. Women, he felt, managed to stay human and in touch with reality, but men grew out of touch with themselves to such an extent that they became as mechanical as the machines and institutions they served. Almost euphorically, he was aware of a changing undercurrent in the Western World. He could only define it as "something more human, more spiritual" trying to surface. Maybe we would have to destroy ourselves completely before we came to our true selves. It was imperative to find a more human way. Maybe with the end of technology, we'd be driven into consciousness? His brain was so seminal that he seemed to take up the space of a crowd. At least in my head. He created that feeling one has when one is a child, that it is all ahead, going to happen, one day.

The medicine man was divorced, Irish style, which meant he was separated from his wife, living alone for a year, but letting on it was to cut down on travel to and from work. Eventually, we decided to live together as consenting adults. Consenting, without the expectation of incessant ever-after happiness, not bound to each other by anything but goodwill and the inevitable challenge. The battle to survive as a whole person while being a woman in relation to a man was as difficult as I had expected. He, in turn, was amazed to discover that I meant it when I said I would not mammy him, or be a wife.

Then in 1977 came my daughter's wedding, my elder son's engagement and departure from home, the removal of my youngest on a musician's tour of somewhere. I was free. I couldn't grasp such freedom, just like that. It was like being in a huge meadow on my own. For the first time since I was nineteen-years-old — no, for the first time in my entire life — I belonged to myself alone, responsible for no one. Nobody to support but me, nobody to feed.

It shook me up, without my even realising why I was shaken. The energy that had kept me bashing away at jobs and home and other activities seemed to ebb suddenly, as if it had a mind of its own and decided "I'll slither off; no longer needed here."

I felt sad, and glad, free, sometimes resentful, abandoned. So this was it; after all those hectic years, I'd made it. The time was mine, my life, my own. Amazing, like one of those dreams in which there's only space. Everything seemed different now, and I questioned my reasons for doing most things.

Empty nest syndrome? You bet. Nest? I felt the urge to fly. I didn't quite know where. Just out. I became impatient with myself, especially spiritually. I wanted to travel, to work at projects rather than a five-day-week job, write books, maybe walk the roads of Ireland from top to bottom. Contemplated staying in bed for a year, but was too restless.

I began by leaving the "Late Late" in 1978. That year Marie McMahon was brought to court on a charge of being a common prostitute. The first I knew of it was when Máirín Johnston rang to ask me to sign a petition and come to the court. Marie's political activism had once again drawn the attention of the powers that be. As well as being a member of the IWLM, Marie, a typesetter with her own business, was in the Irish Civil Rights Association, the editorial committee of *Banshee,* and the Committee for the Abolition of Capital Punishment. She had already been jailed for three months in 1971 for her Vietnam protest, and had previously been involved in the occupation of Hume Street to prevent the demolition of Georgian houses there. In 1977, she'd been arrested under the Emergency Powers Act for putting up posters about a Mansion House meeting against the banning of *Spare Rib.* Some months later, she was again charged with postering "No Heavy Gang, No Torture, No Hanging", which was likely to lead to a breach of the peace.

Now, she had been arrested once again, while walking by the canal with a prostitute. This woman had been on an RTE programme on prostitution presented by Pat Kenny, and she had helped with research. She was arrested by three vice-squad Gardaí, patrolling the area in an unmarked car. Marie was escorting her at the time because she was afraid of meeting her husband, who was rumoured to have returned from England. Marie was charged with prostitution, and using obscene language; a charge of breach of the peace had been dropped.

On a clammy Thursday in July, the Bridewell's No. 6 Court was jammed with supporters. Marie's predicament almost seemed worth while, to bring together so many friends. According to her lawyer, the Gardaí arrested her after yelling: "Hey, you with the hair" which they denied. *They* said she told the garda that she would "fuck him in the canal". Cross-questioning revealed that she had not been told why she was arrested, and only after repeated insistence was shown an ID card. At this point, District Justice Delap dismissed the case, even though the guards protested: "She was so aggressive that we didn't think she would appreciate the reason."

We cheered and applauded, and Justice Delap reprimanded her lawyers over the noise, saying it was illegal to picket a court of law.

A victory, yes, but what of the treatment of our sisters who are kicked about, abused and despised as "common prostitutes" while the men who employ them go publicly guiltless? When I had researched a prostitution story for the "Late Late", I'd hung around a "red light" area for a couple of evenings and was amazed by the fancy cars which drew up to women in the street and did business in time to be home for tea. I wrote some of the licences down, but who would want to know?

1978 was the year I went to California and India. I was jaded when I took off, jolted alive again in a sort of two-part evolution by the trips. Everything there is to say about beautiful bountiful California, where everyone is expected to have at least one dream and all dreams are considered a commitment, has already been said. Anyway, I didn't go in search of copy. I never made a note or stepped out of my way to meet anyone a journalist or feminist ought to meet. And I was living for most of the time among film stars.

And yet I got something of the feel of the place. The thing I first noticed was that even activists didn't talk about women's liberation socially; there weren't those excruciating Irish conversations about rôles and who helped who with the housework. They talked about their work, news, travel, ideas, children. One got the feeling that the new way was accepted, the current reality; I could also see the sadness of some older women for whom it had all come too late, and the confusion of women I met in a professional circle who balked bitterly at being housewives, but hadn't got it together to do anything else. One claimed her liberation in terms of going out to dinner every night or having her husband pick up a takeaway. Why should she be the one to cook? Her new stove gleamed, in her perfect kitchen but it was strictly for show while she fought out her conflict. In the bedroom too, she assured me she had claimed her rights as a person and there was no way she would tolerate lazy behaviour. Her husband seemed puzzled, but kind. I was mortified to be introduced to him as a "liberated woman". He took me aside and asked me how much I earned. Who'd paid for my ticket? Exactly how did I spend my days? For instance, when I got home, what would I do on my first working day? He was having a hard time sorting out what exactly some women had that his wife wanted. She has since set up a thriving business and I like to think of them cooking the evening meal together.

The great thing about California is the atmosphere of acceptance, the freedom to be oneself, the way people say "right on" or "great idea" instead of our "ah sure ..." or "it'll never work ..." It's a validating, highly demanding society, more especially for women, and I was shocked by the materialism, consumerism and outrageous waste. One day I left a restaurant by the wrong door and found myself in the back yard. The food that piled up in the bins and over the yard — big portions of meat, vegetables, pie and bread — was enough to feed an average family for weeks or a small village for a day. "Eyes bigger than their bellies", I thought.

I was also over-awed by the earnestness of Californians, their pursuit of excellence. However, the earnestness had its funny side. For instance, I met a man who was so anxious to improve himself that he was seeing two psychiatrists at the same time, pretending to be faithful to each of them. Then there was the sad story of the hummingbirds, darling little bee-like creatures for whom Californians provide wee bird-houses and food. The birds are accustomed to this source of welfare, depend upon it now. While I was there media announcements warned that they were dropping dead in their thousands because of being fed the sugar substitute "Sweet 'N' Low" by diet-mad Californians.

The best of that trip, for me, was all I learned by living with an Irish couple, Fionnula Flanagan and Garrett O'Connor. Garrett is a psychiatrist who is pioneering revolutionary work in the treatment of alcoholism; he is a friend and colleague of my medicine man. Fionn, whom I had not previously met, also hailed from Dublin. We arrived in Los Angeles two days before her great one-woman show "Joyce's Women" opened downtown. It was written, produced and acted by herself, with Garrett as the sole supporting actor, and Burgess Meredith as director. We rang from our motel and moved in with them after the show opened. It has been all round the world since, including Dublin for James Joyce's centenary celebrations, and has been developed and produced as a film for television by Fionnula and Garrett's Rejoycing Company. The film is to be distributed by Universal Studios.

Although I was bowled over by Fionnula Flanagan's work, the thing which impressed me so profoundly was Garrett and Fionn's marriage, the day-to-day workings of which I couldn't help but see since I lived in their home. A great deal had evolved in the relationship, I could tell, so that now they seemed to have worked out a way of living together in which nobody thought of asking who owed what to whom.

It was never a matter of whose turn it was to do anything. What had to be done was done by whoever was in the house, which happened to be mostly Garrett since Fionn went out to Universal Studios at 6 a.m. most mornings. They seemed to speak so directly and honestly to each other, without undercurrents or manipulation. A tremendous breeze of freedom blew through their house. Anything you wanted to do, not do, think or disagree with was OK. One day I asked Fionn what she thought about my having my face lifted. "It's your face," she said, "if you want it lifted, don't let anyone put you off. If you do decide to get it done, I'll find you someone good. That's important." In Dublin it would have been "oh, don't be silly," or "it doesn't need lifting". Staying in that house taught me that it is possible to live at peace with a man, without being passive or aggressive. It takes a bit of working out, but it does away with destructive games and you wind up as two people living two lives together.

Fionn told me she hadn't always known how she

wanted to live her life. "Then, one day, I said 'I *do* want to be famous, I *do* want to be rich'. So I began to get on with it. We changed things in our lives, but you've got to know the way you want to live your life, and commit yourself to it ..."

India was an utterly different experience. Whereas I loved visiting California, I would gladly live in India for the rest of my life. I've been back there twice since, and will go again as soon as possible. For me, it was more than a discovery of the other side of the world; it brought out the other side of myself, the emergence of my spiritual life which had lain struggling and dormant in my Western life. It gave me a sense of balance within myself which I never would have thought possible.

Not that everyone has to travel to the opposite side of the world to find balance; the journey exists within oneself. I had started it in 1977 when I met a young woman, Bairbre Reddy, in Dublin. She practised Sahaj Marg, a spiritual form of meditation. The system was attractive to me because it seemed to resolve my old conflict with my inherited religions, to go beyond religion to spirituality, and there was no question of rules or regulations I couldn't go along with. I had always had faith, always been a believer, but my religious conflict had made it impossible for me to practice one thing without thinking I was being a traitor to the other. Sahaj Marg solved all that for me, not immediately but eventually.

I went to India to meet the Master of Sahaj Marg, a saintly personality in his eighties, Shri Ram Chandra of Shahjahanpur, Uttar Pradesh, who fondly addressed me as "Sister". If I had felt selfconscious about the whole Indian guru thing before I met him, it was dispelled when I sat in his presence. (A person with similar vibrations is Mother Teresa of Calcutta).

I have never been the same since. "God is not to be found within the fold of a particular religion or sect. He is not confined within certain forms or rituals nor is He to be traced out from within the scriptures," writes Ram Chandra. "Him we have to seek for in the innermost core of our heart." And none of that seeking has led me away from feminism; quite the reverse. If anything, it has confirmed my belief that discrimination of any kind, against anyone, is wicked.

India is unbelievably hospitable. To be fortunate enough to be invited into an Indian home is to know what it is to be treated like beloved visiting royalty. For instance, because I had an Indian friend who had a friend who just happened to have a friend responsible for the gardens of the Taj Mahal, we were given a little cottage on its grounds. As the Muslims and the birds sang in the new day at dawn, I sat in meditation under the bougainvillaea of the Taj gardens, squirrels playing around me, a peacock preening nearby as I closed my eyes.

My friend, Chitra of Agra, even came to the swimming pool with me on the last day. "You are becoming entirely pink," she remarked from her place in the shade, "is that your wish?" It was only in her desire for my happiness that Chitra would ever sit anywhere near a swimming pool in the first place. Feeling foolish and decadent, I explained that I was going to be tanned when the pink faded. She answered, gently; "You are *supposed* to be white." And yet, between us there seemed no reality of different worlds, this world and the Third World, only one world, a world in which we are women together. She is puzzled and vaguely frightened by what she perceives as the life-style of women in my corner of the world. I find it utterly painful and enraging to imagine the reality of most women's lives in India. As in the case of the girl, Shanti. "Shanti is gone," Chitra had answered my inquiry. "How do you mean, gone?" I asked, alarmed for the eleven-year-old girl whom I'd met in India less than three years ago. "She is married," my friend said sadly. Her eyes avoided mine. I remembered that she had wanted to educate this child of her widowed servant, and eventually, to find her a good husband. I had tried to persuade Chitra that Shanti and Chitra's own daughter, now a medical student, must be allowed to choose their own men, even suggested that the girls might remain single. Now Shanti was gone, given in marriage. The child had not wanted it, but "I couldn't interfere too much," explained Chitra, "their caste marry early. It is not possible to make them see. The poor are afraid to change. They do not even know that they are breaking the law ..."

Who would implement the law, anyhow? There are so many laws now to benefit Indian women. There is a law against the dowry system and still women die because of dowry. "Brides are not for burning", "stop atrocities against women", scrawled on walls in Bombay and New Delhi are not slogans of a lunatic fringe. They sent me in search of feminists. This was my second trip to India in three years. I realise now that first trip was spent in the parlour. I fell utterly in love with the beauty, excitement and jumbled consciousness that is India, was delighted by the hospitality and spiritual vitality of the people I met. I was too ready, therefore, to accept answers assuaging the peace of mind of a tourist and the pride of hosts. Of course I saw the poverty, knew of the illiteracy, noted how feverishly people worked for so little, but I was on holiday and for the first time in my adult life, deliberately avoiding contact with media people.

This time, I had no difficulty finding feminists. There are hundreds of old established organisations working for women's rights in India and increasing numbers of militant feminist groups. Neither is there any dearth of organisations of men fighting against social injustices, many of which are specifically related to women. There have been women's progressive movements in India for a century. Now there are third generation feminists. The largest women's organisation, The All India Women's Conference, had as its founder the late Dr. Margaret Cousins, an Irishwoman who fought with the suffragettes in England and Ireland for seven years. She went to India at the request of another Irishwoman, Dr. Annie Besant.

The AIWC was radical in the context of the times and has been responsible for bringing about major changes in legislation which on paper have enormously improved the status of Indian women. This mass of legislation deals with child marriage, prostitution, divorce, property, adoption, working conditions, dowry, and so on. Because of the enormous problems of poverty, many of these organisations have been forced to act in a charitable rather than political capacity, but AIWC has always concentrated on political change while carrying out social and charitable projects. Since the mid-seventies, more militant women's groups have been emerging, one simply called "a group of women", which produces a first-rate bi-monthly magazine in Hindi and English. To give illiterate women a voice, it uses tape recorders in villages at meetings and for personal interviews. These are then translated from the many Indian dialects. In Delhi I met with the feminists who publish *Manushi*, and was reminded, once again that women are a universal class whose sufferings are the result of being born female. Even in India, where one's heart goes out to the poor man trying to eke out a living, one knows that the woman who is dependent upon him has, incredibly, an even crueller life. If only the women's movement in the richer countries could get to the stage of helping our sisters in countries like India.

There are those who'd have us believe that the international women's movement is dead or dying, that it has shot its bolt, and what we are ready for now is an "equality movement". Men, we are told, are ready and willing and able to change the world so that we can take our place in it. Perhaps that time has come for some people. It may have come in America, where Betty Friedan claims in her new book, *The Second Stage*, that feminism demanded an end to women's exploitation within the family, not an end to the family itself. She says that the second stage may not even be a women's movement, but men and women together, and that this stage has to transcend the battle for equal power in institutions. "The second stage will reconstruct the institutions and transform the nature of power itself." It doesn't seem to me to be a stage that has yet arrived in Ireland, nor yet in India. Too much remains to be done before women can work as equals, with or without men.

The women's liberation movement is the great success story of the last decade. Even the recession of the 'eighties, which sent many a woman scurrying back into the "reality" of male economics, has not stopped the growth of feminism. The women's movement in Ireland not only survived the breaking-up of a mass movement before it got off the ground, but feminism became stronger as a result of that breaking-up. Feminism is alive and well and flourishing in Ireland, even though the movement now seems fragmented. There is an established feminist philosophy in the country. Add together the aims of groups and individuals working on single issues, and an overall feminist mandate emerges: control over our bodies and health, equal pay and equal opportunities, equal social welfare service for women, equality before the law, an end to stereotyping in education, an end to stereotyping in the media, the right to self-determined sexuality, an end to violence against women, child-care facilities, recognition of women in the home. Now at last there is a Women's Centre in Dublin's Dame Street, which provides a place for women to meet, share skills, socialise, organise, co-ordinate. It provides a supportive atmosphere for conservative and radical feminists and all shades in between.

The problem with the Irish women's movement during the past few years has been lack of funds; in a time of acute recession there has been less and less money available for anything that might improve women's lot in society. I'm listening for the clamorous baritone sounds of an approaching equality movement, but can't pick up a sound. So we still need the women's movement.

When I emigrated in the 'fifties, or rather when I went to my husband's place of domicile, I didn't even realise how much of a non-person I was as a woman in Irish society. When I came back again in 1965 it was worse, because now I didn't realise I had actually failed at being a non-person. Today, a young Irishwoman has signposts marking her way on almost any road she wishes to take. That type of energy is needed in the continuing life of the Irish women's movement.

EPILOGUE

EPILOGUE:
MOTHER OF THE BRIDE

It was in the summer Nuala ran for election, 1977, that my daughter Diane, aged twenty-two, announced her engagement to James Pilot, an American living in Dublin. They had been attending a Jewish wedding and arrived back around midnight looking vaguely infected and quite delirious. My daughter especially had caught the germ of hysteria, triumph and sheer tribalism which characterises the headiness of the Jewish wedding. Joy knows no bounds. Delight prevails.

"Please God by you," say parents and relatives to each other. "Thank you, I should be so lucky," the recipient of the wish will reply, damp-eyed at the thought of such communal lime-light. Indeed, upon such an occasion it is not unseemly to remark, wistfully, in the vague direction of the Lord: "Please God by me?"

I reflected bitterly that Diane had chosen her time well for announcing: "Pilot and I are getting married." (He has always been called Pilot rather than James). I was sitting with my friends Mannè and Marie Berber, relentless supporters of Tradition, with the obvious exception of pogroms, and quite unable to believe that I did not wish marriage to befall a daughter of mine. With maddening charity, they put my attitude down to my own sad experience of the institution. Now, the noise was incredible, joyous cries of "Mazeltov!" from Marie and one or two others, jumping about, hugging and kissing and "what'll we wear?" and "imagine, it's only yesterday you were this size!" This to a couple who had been living happily together for three years. Mannè chuckled with delight. "You are," he told Pilot, "an extremely lucky man." The well-worn script went on and on, me feeling the urge to walk out in the middle. I glanced at Pilot furiously. "Whoops," he said by way of recognition and darted elsewhere. Now my daughter was standing with her arms around her Uncle Mannè and midst the blushes, wet eyes and bloody nonsense she looked at me around Mannè's beard. She was not surprised at what she saw. Our eyes argued for several seconds and then her eyes said: "It's my life, this is what I'm going to do!"

I moved into the kitchen to make tea, thinking *"Why?"* as if she had said the words aloud. Now at last I understood mothers who asked the demented question: "How could you do this to me?" And again, "where did I go wrong?" Hadn't I done my best to guide her out of the land of bondage?

"Whatever way one desires to go one is led," someone said in the Old Testament. I could, I thought, as I got the cup down, have accepted anything from her but this, this suicidal attempt on her own identity, this turning from the high breezes to the deadening air of the marriage cupboard. This daughter of mine, this sister whose strength, whose sheer female power, so often caused me to smile contentedly, how could she contemplate an about-turn? What could a husband do for her save blur her identity, block her light? What could she expect from marriage that she did not have in abundance within herself? This was the woman who four years earlier had said of a friend who was getting married: "She hasn't an idea who she is yet, but she actually seems to be running away from finding out. That's one of her reasons for getting married, I'm sure."

I felt deeply sad, standing there in the kitchen, thinking about what was happening to my daughter. They'd got her. In spite of all we had experienced about marriage as the place wherein power was most obviously balanced in favour of men, they'd got her. In marriage, we had agreed, women went into service and men were served. Economic helplessness and exhaustion were symptoms of marriage in women. They were drained, depleted, humiliated. Because of the marriage game, women were forced to be manipulative, hypocritical. We had observed that successful marriages were not simply ones that did not end in divorce and separation. There were good marriages, we had agreed, but they were a triumph of humanity over the institution, "in spite of them all". To a woman marriage meant having to ask permission for one's very existence. At least, I thought we'd agreed to all that. And even if we had?

Now I was feeling as if a vital part of myself had been yanked out of its roots, my daughter and myself suddenly such separate beings. How much of her had I sucked within myself, how much had I projected into her? How free had she been that day, in a women's group, when it was decided that the younger and older women separate and she'd wanted me to join her group? "You can't judge by years," she'd said, "I feel more on a wavelength with Mum than girls my own age."

The steam from the kettle was everywhere, the chocolate biscuits on the plate all hazed over, my mind like a March hare's; then I sensed that delicate smell of "L'Air du Temps" and I felt the slender arm around my waist, the silky hair under my cheek. "It'll be all right, Mum, you'll see. Nothing can ever spoil what's between you and me. But we'll have to talk. We've a lot to talk about. And don't blame Pilot, love, it's my idea ..."

We all had tea with lots more noise, and Diane and Pilot left before the Berbers. My throat was tight and stiff, my head ached and when I fell asleep eventually, I dreamed of Diane. But first, before I saw her, I knew I was in hell. Hell was crowded and I knew most of the people and they kept wishing me "Mazeltov" or "Congratulations", and there seemed to be an undercurrent to their wishes, a faint sneer, an insulting knowingness. There was not a single person in that crowded place with whom I could identify in my terrible predicament. It was not clear at first what the predicament was, but I could find no face to accept it, no-one who would listen and hear, no one who would not brush aside how I felt, or change the subject. Everyone else shared something and I was quite, quite alone. My sons, Adam and Michael were there and Adam looked worried, but Mike told him: "The old dear's freakin' out, I'll get her a Crunchie." Then Noelette, Adam's girlfriend from County Clare came and sat down beside me, looking like a young and frightened Edna O'Brien and I moved away from her for fear I'd make her worse. I searched for my mother and could not find her. Nor could I find Diane.

At this point I woke up, wide awake and sweating, and got up and made a cup of tea. I sat and stared into space until it was cool enough to drink and then went back to bed again, fell asleep and found myself immediately in hell again. Everyone was talking and shouting; nobody was saying anything. They all looked pleased and sort of happy and in the centre of all this was a huge golden cage, suspended, swinging from the ceiling and in it, dressed in scanty stage gear, dancing frantically, was my daughter, Diane. The cage kept swinging, the music thumped, the lights flashed in the smoky darkness, everyone went on smiling and Diane kept on dancing. Diane danced for them, even though they hardly seemed aware of her. Dripping sweat, she danced on and on, delighted that everyone was sort of happy. The awful night ended and I awoke to find it was Monday, the off-day from the "Late Late", and I stayed in bed, drifting in and out of sleep, having taken the telephone off the hook after the first call to congratulate me on Diane's engagement.

The dream, had in fact, been tied into a summer that particularly belonged to Diane and myself when she was sixteen. She had gone to the French countryside as an *au pair* to a couple of artists and their children. She hadn't known they were nudists, and when she wrote she told me: "I've got quite used to it now. I'm not careful where I look any more, but I still keep on my bikini." One day, I was in the front room when I heard the gate open. I saw the postman staggering up the path with a heavy parcel. There'd been some parcel bombs in the news and as I opened the door, I said: "I don't know if I should take that, it could be a bomb. Who's it from?"

"Missus," he said, panting and placing the weight on the carpet in front of him, "I don't care if it is a bomb, it weighs a ton and it's costing you a bomb. Payment on delivery from France."

It was a large cement sun-dial made by Diane, carved J—U—N—E when you twisted your head round to read it and it did, indeed, cost a bomb. More than a ten pound note twelve years ago. A letter was enclosed, announcing my daughter's intention to become a sculptor and saying she would probably stay with her artist friends rather than return to school, and perhaps when I decided to visit I'd remember not to bring my usual burden of luggage, since I wouldn't need any clothes, except for going and coming from Ireland. The summer was still young and so was Diane, so I wrote thanking her for the sun-dial and asking her to tell me more. It took a number of letters, before Diane mentioned that she suspected granite sculpting might not be for her after all. I replied, saying I hoped that she had not been tempted to give up too easily. After all, anything worth doing, etc. No word at all from Diane for a couple of weeks, and then a telegram arrived: "Not returning. Staying in Paris to become go-go dancer. Letter following." The letter arrived and I took off to Paris. She was thrilled to see me and she was bubbling over with summertime. She and her friends took me to see go-go dancing. It was in a dark, smoky place with a crowd and lights and thumping music and lovely, almost nude girls dancing in a golden cage.

* * *

When I got my final divorce papers through the post in 1967, I read them carefully and said aloud: "Well, that's one mistake I won't make again." I suspect that my decision to stay in Ireland, a country so hostile to the separated parent and the possibility that she or he be given a second chance at marital disaster, was partly my unconscious insurance against remarriage. I got my divorce by the simple expediency of using the oppressive laws against women to my own advantage. As an Irishwoman living apart from my Canadian husband for three years, I was still domiciled in Canada according to Irish law. Then I would get a divorce in Canada. I had to travel "home" to instigate this, but I never had to appear in court. It was all done by proxy through an Irish solicitor and a Canadian solicitor. But it wasn't divorce that made me want to avoid marriage. It was marriage. Not until the Gaj's group did I begin to work out the knots of that institution, and wonder how I could have been so ignorant of what I was getting into. And now, Diane and I, as she had observed, had so much to talk about.

"Why?"

"You got married," she told me gently and firmly, "I was reared in a marriage. OK, maybe it was unhappy at the end, especially when you got sick, but I remember being happy when I was young here in Ireland and then in my lavender room in Canada. You were different then. I like you as you are now, but I liked you then too. It was a different you for a different time. And you were very feminine and brought me up like that. I had dolls, remember, and tea-sets. I know now there are better toys for children, but I was conditioned in my early years to be traditional. I thought I wasn't the type, but I am."

"You mean there have been no gains made? You've learned *nothing* from ..."

"Look, I don't mean I'm exactly the same as you were. How could I be? But I'm like that in some ways. It seemed nice to me until I was nine."

I sighed, resolving to write this down so that women may know: By watching you your daughter learns what it is to be a woman. You can't tell her which bits to copy. You can't say: "cancel that bit, I didn't realise you were watching, I've changed my mind."

Diane said: "I'm getting married to please myself. The time has come to get married. The time will come to have children. There'll be times for different things in our relationship. Now it's marriage."

"What is the difference between being married and

living together?"

"I'll tell you when I know. But I'm doing what I want, not what people expect or to get out of anything. I'm not patriarchy's woman, and Pilot's as much a feminist as you are, as you well know."

"What about your ambitions and goals, your love of travel?"

"Ah come on now, you sound like something out of the Ark!"

"Whose job will be given up when children arrive?" I insisted. "Probably neither, except for a short time, but the way this society is run I'll probably be the one who gets to mind the baby. Poor Pilot won't have the chance."

The talks went on. One night she wafted a diamond ring under my nose, saying: "I know how you feel, but isn't it lovely?" Now it was official. Meanwhile, I had started telling people, feeling confused. I was happy she was happy, happy she was doing her own thing, but frightened for her life. Now the full uproar was growing like a mushroom under my nose: family guest lists — a small wedding, but we've a huge family — dates, honeymoon brochures, arguments. It was like a driving wind at my back. But there were some women who understood how I felt, which was a comfort.

"You," Diane said over a meal together one night, "are fighting against the independence you taught me. Y'see, in your day people may have just gone into marriage blindly because they didn't know any other way. I'm not getting married because it's inevitable. It's not the only or the best trade open to me. I have my career. I'm not going to copy anyone else's marriage. You think I'm being sucked in by the system. I'm not. Not any system. I'm my own person. We are getting married," said Diane, "not so he becomes my breadwinner and I become his housekeeper. If people want to live like that, maybe it suits them. We can both cook, sew, change fuses, paint, garden, fill in forms, use a hammer and nails, earn our own living. So why would we break off into halves? There are two lives."

Another time, she said: "All the stuff we've talked

about together, all I understand about the sort of marriage I want, I've learned from you in this two-tiered way."

I had assumed they would be married in a registry office since neither came from a religious background. Diane wanted a religious ceremony. I could understand that, but the thought of going into an orthodox synagogue to endure the male power trip was something from which I cringed. In the home, the Jewish woman may manage to accept herself as "more precious than rubies ...", her official image, so to speak, since the days of King Solomon, but in the synagogue her value is less obvious. It is not all that different from a Hindu temple, Muslim mosque or Christian Church, but at least in the latter a female is obliged to attend and receives Holy Communion. I recall my surprise on one Sabbath, as a child, when I found myself standing beside a woman who prayed earnestly all through the service. The other women chatted, returning to their prayer books sometimes, not seeming involved in the purpose of being there. So, there they'd be, the men, circumcised and barmitzvahed, their prayer shawls around their shoulders, their yamikas (skull caps) in place, all set to conduct the day's business with their God. Like so many spiders weaving a web around my Diane. Then there would be the reception, with speeches from men in their pride, as if women hadn't a tongue in their heads.

It didn't happen that way. Diane may be "conservative", but she dreads being a hypocrite. She wanted to start her Jewish marriage as she meant to go on; therefore she decided that the Liberal or Reform way of Judaism would better suit her ability to practise it. She and Pilot began attending the liberal synagogue. Joan Finkel, whose father had founded the synagogue, helped them to become members and have their wedding there. Diane said it was a joy to "do business" with both sexes of a synagogue, to feel one could be a real part of it, to enjoy such a free atmosphere. She had always loved the spirit of Judaism, been irritated with its rigidity, and looked forward to a wedding in English, "a ceremony that will mean something to Pilot and me."

On the one hand, I still wished it wasn't happening, but on the other, I had now become The Mother Of The Bride. Maybe getting obsessive about the wedding day was a way of avoiding my feelings of loss, of threat, of jealousy of one James Pilot. What, I kept asking myself, had he done to deserve his luck?

So I trudged around looking at wedding dresses and honeymoon gear. Glazed looks came across the faces of young women with whom I worked when I went on about what to wear, but I couldn't seem to stop. Part of it all was that I had developed a case of regression. As I busied myself with Diane's wedding, the time of my own marriage replayed in my head. I peeled off tons of weight, had facials, manicures, lived for the day. But after I'd decided what to wear, ordered the cake and completed the lists, I sort of froze up. I didn't go and see Joan Finkel to consult about final arrangements. I kept putting it off. There was a lull. Then one evening Diane arrived, with Pilot, to announce: "Rabbi Julia is doing the ceremony: She'll come for the week-end."

"Rabbi who?" I asked, knowing I'd heard wrong. "Did you say *she?*"

"Sure," Diane said, grinning, "I've got a woman rabbi, Rabbi Julia Neuberger from England. She's the first woman Rabbi in this part of the world ..." I was bawling. Such a possibility had never even occurred to me. It changed everything: "Rabbi Julia! Rabbi Julia!" I kept repeating.

The Liberal Synagogue hadn't got a resident rabbi, and when Diane discovered there was a woman rabbi in England she asked Joan to engage her for the wedding. The rabbi said she could not come on that date; the date could not be changed. Diane rang Rabbi Julia asking her to come somehow, explaining how much it would mean to her and "my mother" to have a female rabbi perform the ceremony. Rabbi Julia was coming. Or Rabbi Neuberger as everyone else properly called her.

Now, there were murmurings about "giving the bride away". God, what primitive rubbish, I grumbled. How could anyone give away what they did not own? I had reared her, loved her, into my care she had been given, but I had never *owned* her. She was not mine to give and if not mine then whom else's? Had her father been around I would have suffered him to lead her up the aisle for both their sakes, but in his absence? It was suggested discreetly that it was her grandfather's place, or her eldest brother's. I was not sure how this could be avoided, for although in the strict sense Jewish brides are not given away, they are usually led up the aisle by a male relative. Diane found a solution: "Can Mum do it," she asked Joan Finkel, "can Mum walk up the aisle with me?"

"I can't think why not," was the reply.

Meanwhile, the orthodox Berbers were standing up, in the Liberal Synagogue, for Pilot whose father was dead and whose mother was unable to travel. The wedding was on Sunday, and on the Saturday the Sabbath Service, with the bridal couple attending, was conducted by Rabbi Julia before everyone went back to lunch at the Berbers. Seeing Rabbi Julia stand in front of the Ark, handle the Holy Scrolls of Moses, leader among all those men in black, I glanced at Marie to see how she was taking it. She was grinning from ear to ear.

I spent some time, over lunch, chatting with Rabbi Julia, in her late twenties, at most barely thirty, married, with small children. She had an easy, womanly strength, joy never far from the surface of her awareness, though quiet. She had always wanted to be a rabbi, she told me, always, ever since she used to go to synagogue with her father in London's East End every Saturday morning. She denied that it had been a hard fight to become a rabbi. Somebody had to be first with everything and the drive felt so natural from within herself. She said some of her congregation found it strange, but more and more people were saying: "Why not?" She and her husband shared the family responsibilities, she told me. It was entirely possible to have a really Jewish home with all the effort that implied, even if the wife and mother happened to be a rabbi.

The wedding day came at last, and so did the white Rolls-Royce I had ordered to transport us to the synagogue. My sons fell about laughing at the sight of it. Diane wore a cob-web fine dress of antique Irish lace, from Deirdre Ryan's famous collection of antique Irish handwork (mostly made in the convents of Ireland). I wore pale gold crochet and one of those stabbing ice-cream pains in my right eye. When we got to the synagogue, the mixed choir was already singing. I'd never heard female voices in a synagogue before. We waited, in a little room. "It's nice here," I told Diane, "I hope they won't call us too quickly."

It was time. A man, all fuss, came to usher us into the synagogue. Diane put her hand on my arm as we moved to "Here Comes the Bride". Her face was glowing under the veil, her hand felt unnatural where it was. I took it in my left hand, holding it firmly as we walked. The hand had changed since I'd taken my little girl shopping in Dublin city. It was no mere splodge of softness in mine. Soft, yes, but firm and slender, aware, and just as trusting. As we approached the canopy, bedecked with flowers, the rest of the wedding party stood waiting around Rabbi Julia, who looked up from her prayer-book with a soft smile. The sun shone through her golden red hair, curled around a black beret to match her black suit, her skin transparent. We stepped together up under the wedding canopy, still holding hands. I loosened my grasp and Diane's hand slipped away, naturally.

"Diane and Pilot," Rabbi Julia began.